CORRELATIVE URINALYSIS

The Body Knows Best

M.T. Morter, Jr., B.S., M.A., D.C.

Edited by John M. Clark, D.C.

B.E.S.T. Research Inc.
Rogers, Arkansas 72756

Copyright © 1987 by B.E.S.T. Research Inc.

Printed in the United States

Library of Congress Cataloging-in-Publication Data
Morter, M.T.
        Correlative urinalysis.

        Bibliography: p.
        1. Nutrition.   2. Urine—Analysis.   3. Nutritionally induced diseases.   4. Fluid-electrolyte balance.
5. Chiropractic.   I. Clark, John M,   II. Title.
[DNLM: 1. Diet—adverse effects.   2. Urine—analysis.
QV 185 M887c]
RA784.M627 1988   613.2   87-51116
ISBN   0-944994-00-8

. . . Discovery consists of seeing what everybody has seen
and thinking what nobody has thought.

Albert Szent-Gyoergyi

ACKNOWLEDGEMENTS

Talking about "writing a book" is one thing, but actually transforming information into a form that is ready for printer and reader requires the cooperation of a small army of people. First and foremost of these in the preparation of this book has been Dr. John M. Clark, my professional associate and, more important, my long-time friend who tended to the day-to-day process of compiling, researching, organizing and editing the thoughts and concepts into the material you are about to read.

A list complete enough to acknowledge all of the people who contributed to this book's coming into being would take on the proportions of a telephone directory. The seeds for this work were sown by the thousands of patients over the years who have come to me for help in solving a variety of physical problems. Without these patients and the challenges they presented, the research and study that has gone into reevaluating and understanding the wondrous workings of the perfect creation we term "the body" would not have come about. In addition, the material contained in these pages has been shared in nearly 200 seminars with hundreds of Doctors of Chiropractic, many of whom have encouraged me to bring together the information as a unified reference work. To these many friends, patients and supporters, my heartfelt thanks.

Also, to Dr. Dan Roberts and the rest of my clinic and B.E.S.T. staffs, my appreciation for their conscientious attention to the myriad details of serving our patients that makes it possible for me to continue research and study into how the body functions.

Of course, a creative production of any size is a family affair, and my family has not only contributed moral support and encouragement but also cooperated in a professional capacity as consultants, advisors and a collective knowledgeable sounding board. Sons Dr. Ted Morter, Dr. Tom Morter, and daughter, Dr. Sue Morter have all listened to and constructively challenged Dad's theories and conclusions. But it is my wife and best friend, Marjorie, who is "the wind beneath my wings." She has, with her active fertile mind and boundless energy, helped to fine-tune and hone ideas and concepts, develop and stage seminars, devise and produce written, audio and visual materials, and take care of the many administrative functions of B.E.S.T. all the while maintaining a warm, cheerful, welcoming home. To Marjorie goes a special thanks.

CONTENTS

TABLES, LISTS, AND CHARTS

FOREWORD

Dr. Morter has succeeded in reducing the complexity of biochemistry to a few salient points: (1) Dr. Morter believes that the American diet is too high in protein. The goal should be an input of 41 grams of protein, or, perhaps, even less. He claims that increased acidity of the body and an accumulation of ammonia is the result of protein. The combination of increased acidity and increased ammonia levels leads the body to become susceptible to viruses, yeast infections, and even pain. (2) Dr. Morter also espouses the view that the best diet is a diet that consists of fruits and vegetables which tend to make the body more alkaline so that the urinary pH approaches 7.5.

The idea that protein should be restricted to 41 grams or less is one that is certainly appealing. People have long suspected that it is not only protein but the fat associated with it that is responsible for cardiovascular disease and also for some kinds of cancer. For example, the British medical journal *Lancet* published a study in which it was demonstrated that people who ate a diet high in fruits and vegetables had a lower incidence of abdominal cancer than those who did not. Other studies that identify environmental toxins as being the culprits in carcinogenesis are too numerous to mention. A classical study reported that Japanese women who live in Japan have a very low incidence of breast cancer. When they move to the United States, the incidence of breast cancer increases, presumably an increase that is correlated with the increase of hamburgers in the diet. The idea that protein may be responsible for increasing urinary ammonia is novel; one that I have supported with my research. As the physician in charge of a spinal cord injury center, I became very concerned with the fact that many of my patients were on antibiotics for years (due to bladder infections), and they had lost a significant amount of muscle mass. I began doing amino acid analysis in both plasma and urine in order to find some clue as to why they were losing their muscle mass. To my surprise, not only did the patients show deficiencies in some amino acids but, in many cases, they also showed huge increases in urine ammonia levels. Whereas the normal level was 0-50 mg/ml, some of the patients showed up to 16,000-20,000 mg/ml. Dr. Morter suggests that these ammonia levels are the result of a high protein diet.

Is Dr. Morter right? I started monitoring the pH of the urine of my patients over several months. Most of them had a urinary pH of 6. In cases where it was higher, the increased pH was due to the accumulation of ammonia. In three cases of patients who had levels of ammonia, the levels were brought down within a few days by giving them cranberry juice. We used cranberry juice because it is the only substance that can be ingested by mouth that remains acidic. The acid in the cranberry juice causes the ammonia to become ammonium so that it can be released safely from the body. The patients not only felt better, but they were also able to start on a diet that was more conducive to health. There is no doubt that cranberry juice, given in the right circumstances, acts as an analgesic!

Dr. Morter's focus on urinary pH represents a very common sense approach. Laboratory tests are notoriously inaccurate, expensive, and belated. When you are trying to improve health by monitoring daily fluctuations, laboratory tests are no longer appropriate. Measuring salivary and urinary pH using litmus paper is a simple, inexpensive alternative for detecting the patients' reactions to different dietary regimens.

Judith B. Walker, M.D., Ph.D.
Director of Medicine
Walker Institute
Pacific Palisades, California

TO THE READER

This book has been written to provide practical information about interpreting urinalysis findings to uncover valuable clues that indicate how dietary habits are affecting the body. The following chapters also provide fresh insight into nutrition that will assist doctors in guiding patients through the current maze of misinformation on the subject. They explain factors in physiological relationships that have been overlooked by other researchers which, in turn, led them to arrive at some incomplete conclusions. The research findings and observations cited are from readily available texts.

The material presented here may not agree with currently accepted medical opinion, nor is it intended to explain medical practice pertaining to nutrition. The conclusions and opinions expressed are based on research, careful study, analysis, and twenty-five years of clinical experience. As investigations into the premises set forth in this book continue, observations and findings pertaining to these premises by other scientific and academic researchers are not only welcomed but encouraged.

No endorsement of any particular product brand of supplementation is intended; many fine brands are available. The clinical results described in this book were obtained using the products mentioned.

It is assumed that those using the corrective procedures suggested in this book are trained in the Bio Energetic Synchronization Technique (B.E.S.T.). This is not meant to imply that other chiropractic techniques will not be successful but only to state that the clinical results cited were obtained in conjunction with B.E.S.T.

Practitioners who incorporate the treatment methods discussed in this book are reminded that in the event unfavorable circumstances arise during the course of treatment, it is recommended that a complete and detailed diagnosis be made by another qualified physician, i.e., chiropractor, osteopath, or medical doctor. Regardless of the specialty, the consultant should be trained in holistic health care that will better enable him to understand the intricate relationship between diet and health. The author assumes no responsibility for any negative effects from following the recommendations in this book.

Throughout this book, the masculine gender has been used in order to avoid unwieldy phrases that could detract from the subject matter being discussed. This is strictly a device to advance the flow of the material and is in no way intended to reflect that either patients or doctors are males only.

All dietary changes should be under the direction of a qualified physician.

M.T. Morter, Jr., B.S., M.A., D.C.

1

INTRODUCTION

INVESTIGATING RESPONSES TO TREATMENT

Most doctors who have been in practice for several years have had the experience of seeing a patient in severe pain, yet the patient's x-rays reveal no pathology. Or, conversely, an x-ray may show a tertiary scoliosis and arthritis, but the patient complains merely of an occasional headache. In either case, the patient's symptoms just don't agree with the x-rays. Similarly, the results of urinalysis often appear to totally contradict the symptoms the patient describes; again, the technology and the expressed symptoms don't agree. B.E.S.T. clarifies the x-ray dilemma; the information in this book resolves the issue of apparently disjunctive urinalysis results and correlates the relationship of diet and nutrition with urinalysis findings.

My concentrated investigation into the connection between nutrition and the general well-being of patients was prompted by my observations of the significant variations in patient response to adjustments. As I began to correlate diet with these responses, I assumed that those patients who "ate well" — followed the Standard American Diet (SAD) of a balance of the four basic food groups outlined by the USDA — would respond to treatment more favorably than did those who followed the modern regimen of a fast-food, junk food diet.

However, contrary to my expectations, the results of my clinical investigations indicated that those patients who ate "junk food" responded better to adjustments than did those who ate the SAD. Based on this experience, I concluded that a factor of the Standard American Diet was responsible for the delayed response to treatment of some patients. However, I could not in good conscience recommend that my patients replace the steak, eggs, and milk in their diets with pizza, doughnuts and cola drinks.

There was, from my point of view at that time, no defined reason why those who ate pizza rather than steak should be more responsive to treatment. The steak and potatoes diet, like the chips and dips diet, contained some empty calories, but the primary difference was in the amount of meat — animal protein — consumed. My tentative conclusions ran contrary to the long-standing general conviction that meat is the cornerstone of good nutrition. There was growing evidence that excess dietary protein was the culprit.

Yet, generations of Americans have been schooled in the merits of conscientiously following well-balanced diets of steak, chicken, ham, eggs, cheese, milk, and enriched bread. Concerned parents and grandparents deplore the eating habits of many of today's Americans — pizza, fiber-added-hamburgers, chips, doughnuts, soft drinks, and processed foods.

To resolve this conflict between our cultural traditions and my observations, I undertook extensive clinical and academic research to determine why the Standard American Diet should fare so poorly in my initial comparative study. Over ten years of investigation has not only shown me why our protein-rich diets can produce negative results but it has also greatly reinforced my conviction that the body is governed by a self-healing, self-regulating, self-organizing mechanism. The healing-regulating-organizing is not accomplished by a vitamin, drug, knife, or adjustment — it is brought about by the body itself. It is attributable to a superintelligence that is perfect at all times.

The response of this superintelligence to a stimulus is always perfect. Our responsibilities as doctors are to evaluate and to understand the stimulus in order to determine why the response is necessary. A particular response may not always be Normal — it is often not Natural — but any response by the body is always Necessary.

The urinalysis provides us with the most convenient and reliable means of finding how the body is responding and why a certain response is necessary. It can also give us an accurate method of monitoring any change that takes place.

Many doctors, especially chiropractors, do not utilize urinalysis as a diagnostic aid; perhaps this is justified. Both the analysis findings and the suggested methods of treatment can be confusing. Treatment that seems to work for one patient will have no effect on the second and may make a third patient worse. Rather than trying to reconcile these outcomes, the analysis procedures are often ignored.

Blood tests, although more widely used, cannot equal the diagnostic value of urinalysis in determining a patient's state of health. By the time a blood test shows abnormal findings, the cells and interstitial fluid have already been affected. This can confirm that the patient is ill, but urinalysis can show either positive or negative progression of the state of health.

Nothing occurs in the body independently — stimuli affect cells, tissue, organs and systems — and in our discussions of the various aspects of urinalysis, several topics overlap: protein and pH are closely associated; dietary ash, acidity, and alkalinity have an interwoven relationship; and saliva pH is affected by the same buffering systems that affect interstitial pH. This intertwining of information serves to illustrate even further that the body is one synchronous entity.

THE ORIGINS OF ILLNESS

Despite the thousands of disease names medicine has given us, there are only three reasons why people ever get sick. The first is autointoxication — *toxicity* — which comes from the consumption of food inappropriate for our bodies. Our bodies do not know how to handle this inappropriate food in a normal physiological way, consequently, processing these substances interferes with homeostasis — drugs are an extreme example of this.

The second cause of disease is interference with *timing*. This interference causes impaired internal communication within the individual. Every part of the body is supposed to be synchronized with every other part of the body at all times. If the body's timing is not synchronized, as with an automobile engine, good fuel can be put into it but it will not function at full capacity.

The manner in which the stomach functions is a good example of the critical importance of timing. Hydrochloric acid (HCl) is secreted by the parietal cells when protein is introduced into the stomach. This is a natural response that is vital to the digestion of protein. If, however, HCl is secreted when the stomach is empty, a timing problem exists that will lead to the development of an ulcer. The stomach is doing its job perfectly, but it is doing it at the wrong time and is not coordinated with the rest of the body.

The third cause of disease is *thoughts*. We know that a well-nourished and well-timed body can become ill through habitually negative thoughts. It doesn't make any difference what the thoughts are if they are negative — even an obsession with health can be detrimental if it interferes with the body's built-in drive to health. I term this process subcortical automaticity, meaning that the body responds without conscious thought directing it. Any obsessive cortical activity will interfere with this natural subcortical automaticity.

Our clinical experience shows that the average patient who comes into the office today is suffering from a combination of all three of these factors. Therefore, today's doctor should not only be aware of the multiplicity of the situation but should do everything in his power to correct any or all causes of illness — timing, toxicity, or thoughts. Health is automatic if timing, toxicity and thoughts are corrected. That is why this book is intended to be available to any doctor who is interested in helping his patients achieve total health. It will act as a guide through the maze of contradictory information that assaults us from every side, and it will clarify aspects of health and diet heretofore hazy and obfuscated.

OUR RESPONSIBILITY FOR HEALTH

Most of the physical ills of our society brought about by toxicity are directly related to our diet. Although my early survey indicated that patients on the modern-day junk food diet responded more quickly to adjustments, they too, for the most part, were toxic and trudging unwittingly down the path to chronic degenerative disease. The difference between them and those on the Standard American Diet was that the junk food eaters were moving more slowly down this health-declining road.

We can develop a clear picture of the type of food Americans eat by looking at the items on supermarket shelves and reviewing the menus of most restaurants. In many supermarkets, fresh produce, which should make up approximately 75% of our diet, is at a premium while sugary snacks and processed munchies are prominently displayed throughout the store. And the fare offered by many restaurants is little better. While more and more restaurants offer salad bars as a concession to weight-conscious, health-conscious customers, many menu meals include few, if any, vegetables with the meat and potatoes. Often, a small "salad" of tired lettuce and perhaps a tomato, or a token serving of cole slaw, is the only edible greenery available.

Many Americans consider that following government recommendations concerning the types of foods most beneficial to them will assure good health. Unfortunately, experience illustrates the folly of looking for leadership from those whose status and positions are governed by economics. One of the most blatant illustrations of how economic forces influence governmental policies at the expense of the best interests of the public occurred in 1977.

In February of that year, a publication entitled "Dietary Goals for the United States" was prepared by the staff of the Select Committee on Nutrition and Human Needs, United States Senate. The Foreword by the chairman of the committee, Senator George McGovern (South Dakota), reads, in part: "If we as a Government want to reduce health costs and maximize the quality of life for all Americans, we have an obligation to provide practical guides to the individual consumer as well as set national dietary goals for the country as a whole."[1]

The committee set forth the following suggestions for changes as a means of meeting the newly established dietary goals.

The Goals Suggest the Following Changes in Food Selection and Preparation[2]

1. Increase consumption of fruits and vegetables and whole grains.

2. Decrease consumption of meat and increase consumption of poultry and fish.

3. Decrease consumption of foods high in fat and partially substitute poly-unsaturated fat for saturated fat.

4. Substitute non-fat milk for whole milk.

5. Decrease consumption of butterfat, eggs and other high cholesterol sources.

6. Decrease consumption of sugar and foods high in sugar content.

7. Decrease consumption of salt and foods high in salt content.

Item 1 is highly significant — increase consumption of fruits and vegetables and whole grains. However, the most startling recommendation of this list is Item 2. Decrease consumption of meat and increase consumption of poultry and fish. This recommendation of the committee, prompted by reports on nutrition and health by respected members of the scientific community, is contrary to our cultural trend toward more and more meat consumption. Yet it indicates that nutritionists are becoming increasingly aware of the detrimental effects of excess meat and dairy products.

This booklet was produced in February 1977 and was available for purchase from the U.S. Government Printing Office. However, shortly after publication, this booklet was withdrawn from sale and is no longer available anywhere. However, in December of the same year — ten months later — it was reissued with some significant changes. The December issue gave an expanded and revised seven item list under the same title: "The Goals Suggest the Following Changes in Food Selection and Preparation."[3] However, this list is significantly different. Most items have been watered down, and the recommendation to decrease meat consumption per se has been eliminated. The revised version reads:

1. Increase consumption of fruits and vegetables and whole grains.

2. Decrease consumption of refined and other processed sugars and foods high in such sugars.

3. Decrease consumption of foods high in total fat, and partially replace saturated fats, whether obtained from animal or vegetable sources, with poly-unsaturated fats.

4. Decrease consumption of animal fat, and choose meats, poultry and fish which will reduce saturated fat intake.

5. Except for young children, substitute low-fat and non-fat milk for whole milk, and low-fat dairy products for high fat dairy products.

6. Decrease consumption of butterfat, eggs and other high cholesterol sources. Some consideration should be given to easing the cholesterol goal

for pre-menopausal women, young children and the elderly in order to obtain the nutritional benefits of eggs in the diet.

7. Decrease consumption of salt and foods high in salt content.

Item 1 remained unchanged. No one (and no lobby) will argue about encouraging consumers to buy more of foods as obviously beneficial to health as vegetables and fruit. However, no longer was it recommended that we decrease meat consumption, and all of the other recommendations, except Item 7 concerning salt consumption, have been qualified. It would appear from these changes that only the salt industry is without an effective lobby.

Included in the study is a statement of Dr. Beverly Winikoff, Rockefeller Foundation, New York, concerning the consequences of nutrition-related diseases. Dr. Winikoff stated: "There is a widespread and unfounded confidence in the ability of medical science to cure or mitigate the effects of such diseases once they occur. Appropriate public education must emphasize the unfortunate but clear limitations of current medical practice in curing the common killing diseases. Once hypertension, diabetes, arteriosclerosis of heart disease are manifest, there is, in reality, very little that medical science can do to return a patient to normal physiological function. As awareness of this limitation increases, the importance of prevention will become all the more obvious."[4]

This statement points out the importance of each of us accepting the responsibility for our own health and that of young members of our families. We can meet this responsibility best by becoming aware of how foods affect the body as a whole, and by understanding that the body responds perfectly, every time, to stimuli.

THE BODY DOESN'T KNOW HOW TO BE SICK!

The body never makes a mistake! Never! The body never has to think about what to do — it automatically knows what to do as a response to any stimulus. The body doesn't think. It doesn't think health and it doesn't think disease. It only responds to stimuli and the response is always perfect for the particular stimulus. Our obligation as doctors is to interpret the stimulus correctly, then we will understand the response. If a patient is not happy with a response he gets, he must change the stimulus. That is what this book is all about. We will show you how to change the stimulus. We will also show you how rapidly this change can be made without the patient reverting to his old habits because he felt so bad right after he started the "good" diet you recommended. At the same time, the patient must change his diet just as quickly as possible in order to overcome whatever disease process is being manifest.

It is our intention to help you to understand why one analysis finding shows up along with another that appears to be totally antithetical. We will present the findings, the reasons for the variations in readings, the relationships among systems and processes, the role nutrition plays in our physiological well-being, and finally, we will give suggestions for correcting deleterious situations and for helping your patients achieve or regain their own maximum degree of health. To accomplish this purpose, we must first review briefly some basic physiology and biochemistry that will lay the groundwork for our venture into urinalysis.

2

CONCEPTS AND ASSUMPTIONS

OVERVIEW

This chapter will be a potpourri of elements that are fundamental to understanding the concepts set forth in this book. We will touch on some of the basics of digestion, assimilation, and elimination; define and discuss physiological ash and its relationship to health; and lay the groundwork for investigating the topics in the chapters that follow.

Perhaps most important, we will establish some relationships between biochemistry and physiology that, to my knowledge, have not previously been clearly identified. For example, in his *Textbook of Medical Physiology*, Guyton states that only slight changes in pH will significantly affect the function of the cell[1], yet Cantarow and Schepartz in their *Biochemistry* give normal pH values of gall bladder bile as 5.5 to 7.7.[2] I must accept both of these statements as true; however, they are inconsistent; pH 5.5 to 7.7 allows for considerably more than a "slight change." One of my objectives is to untangle conflicting statements and reduce confusion surrounding the use of urinalysis findings.

In this book, we look at various segments of the interrelationship of several elements of urinalysis. In order to set the stage for our discussion, we will present four basic assumptions that underlie this work.

FIRST ASSUMPTION: THE CONCEPT OF NATURAL, NORMAL AND NECESSARY

The first assumption deals with the concept of Natural, Normal and Necessary — a central theme throughout this material that is essential to understanding the basis for my conclusions and recommendations. "Natural" responses of the body are those that occur when the body operates under natural internal control without having to adapt to adverse circumstances such as those imposed by eating food that has long-range negative impact.

"Normal" refers to those conditions that exist among the majority of people who appear to be asymptomatic. For instance, urine pH of 4.50 to 8.40 is considered normal since this is the range exhibited by most apparently healthy individuals. Actually, the term "average" would be more appropriate than "normal"; under optimal conditions, the urine pH would naturally fluctuate within a rather narrow range from slightly acid to neutral to slightly alkaline. However, since the diets of most Americans consist predominantly of protein-rich foods, out of necessity urine pH varies within the wide range considered normal. The body is impeccably intelligent; it will adapt in order to compensate for unfavorable stresses.

"Necessary" indicates adaptations (often causing discomfort, fatigue, and mental distress) that are required for survival, and if the stimuli that make the adaptations necessary are not changed, chronic degenerative disease will ultimately follow. *The body will respond on a priority basis to do whatever is necessary for it to continue to function* — the body does not know how to be sick.

SECOND ASSUMPTION: THE BODY NEVER MAKES A MISTAKE

Regardless of philosophical viewpoint, most doctors can accept our second assumption that the human body is the ultimate perfection of nature — that the body is created and maintained by some intelligence far greater than that of man.

The alternative to this view is that the body constantly makes mistakes and needs correction — that the body is not intelligent and cannot take care of itself without the assistance of the technologies of man in the form of medication or supplementation. This view is illogical; the body does not make mistakes — perfection is built in! The very best any doctor can do is to assist this marvelous machine to do what it was designed to do. We must learn to listen to its subtle communications and to interpret them. The body's intelligence will not shout, but it will communicate.

Apparently, a philosophy of dual physiology has developed concerning the body's reaction to health and disease. The body does not have one neurological or hormonal network for normal physiology and another network to handle disease. The same organs, glands, and systems that keep our bodies functioning smoothly are the ones that must adapt their responses to interferences brought about by improper diet or other stress-inducing conditions. The response is appropriate to the stimulus, and the human body will respond as best it can to that stimulus. We need to discard dualistic thinking and understand that everything the body does is intelligent and represents its very best effort to survive in the hostile environment to which it is subjected. The body does not know how to be sick — what it does know is how to accommodate, within limits, to abuses that are either consciously or unconsciously inflicted upon it.

If we choose not to accept the assumption that the body is comprehensively intelligent and functions naturally while making minor adjustments, we can spend our lives in a frantic effort to patch one ailment after another while all the time the body continues to deteriorate. This interpretation presupposes some degree of biological stupidity that must be corrected by external intervention such as administering a pill or an injection, or by removing a malfunctioning organ. It is easy to see why the medical doctor would accept this view when he can see dramatic improvement in the patient's comfort (if not digestion) following removal of the gall bladder. This apparent contradiction of our assumption that the body never makes a mistake will be resolved in the discussion of bilirubin in Chapter Six.

THIRD ASSUMPTION: THE "REALITY" OF SCIENCE

Our third assumption is that medical science is made up of a generally accepted compilation of opinions, theories and conclusions that are a synthesis of scientific research, experimentation and experience. The information presented in this book is also the result of research and clinical experience. Although the conclusions differ markedly in many instances from those currently expressed by medical science, it should be remembered that ongoing scientific findings continually alter well-established hypotheses. One of my purposes in presenting this material is to offer a carefully considered point of view concerning causes of illness in order that these premises may act as a catalyst for research efforts of others.

In an article entitled "Is There Such A Thing As Scientific Objectivity?" in the September 1985 edition of *Discover* magazine,[3] K.C. Cole makes the point that there is no such thing as scientific fact. Most of us prefer to think of science as being cut and dried, exact, and thoroughly predictable. Unfortunately, science is not this way.

Cole quotes science historian Paul Feyerabend as saying: "... we even find that science knows no 'bare facts' at all, but that all the 'facts' that enter our knowledge are already viewed in a certain way." All too often, the scientist finds facts to substantiate what he has already accepted. In the same article, Thomas Kuhn, Massachusetts Institute of Technology science historian, is quoted as referring to scientific research as "a strenuous and devoted attempt to force nature into the conceptual boxes supplied by professional education." Kuhn goes on to say, "In science . . . novelty emerges only with difficulty, manifested by resistance, against a background provided by expectation. Initially, only the anticipated and usual are experienced even under circumstances where anomaly is later to be observed." The message conveyed is that scientific objectivity is inevitably blurred by the biases built into human perception. The true measure of scientific objectivity is consensus. When sufficient numbers of scientists agree, a premise is accepted as fact.

This is both good and bad. Acknowledging the essential subjectivity of science makes it stronger by keeping the door open to interpretation. Accepting a single objective truth, on the other hand, means that some day that door will be closed. Cole also cites Feyerabend as writing, "Unanimity of opinion may be fitting for a church, for the frightened or greedy victims of some (ancient or modern) myth, or for the weak and willing followers of some tyrant. . . . Variety of opinion is necessary for objective knowledge."

The observations presented in this book are based on the cumulative results of over a decade of intensive search and research to find answers to questions that came to my mind years ago. During this time only procedures that I found worked 100% of the time were incorporated into my technique. If a procedure failed once, it was discarded.

My approach to nutrition was no less exacting but certainly much more difficult in that I had to wade through a vast swamp of misinformation. Yet here and there I found a nugget of truth. Eventually, I found enough of these to form my theories. Perhaps the information presented here is not new in the sense of discovery, but it is certainly new in its interpretation. In Cole's article he quotes Albert Szent-Gyoergyi: "Discovery consists of seeing what everybody has seen and thinking what nobody has thought."

Some authoritative views and conclusions are based on an inaccurate premise. In *Harper's Review of Biochemistry*, the statement is made that it is normal for the body to excrete 16.5 grams of nitrogen per day.[4] This amount is predicated on the assumption that individuals consume 100 grams of protein per day. The remainder of the chapter as well as other related parts of the book are valid for persons who consume this amount. However, 100 grams per day is between five and ten times more protein than the body can effectively handle. This means that all subsequent conclusions regarding protein metabolism are true based upon a daily consumption of 100 grams of protein yet these same conclusions must be called into question if the daily intake of protein is reduced to 10 to 20 grams — the level at which the body was designed to function naturally.[5]

We have seen that the scientific findings of each research project and experiment, whether laboratory or clinical, are subject to interpretation of the researcher who, like the rest of us, is confined by human limitations of current knowledge. It is not my intention to discount medical science and research — much of the background information presented here has been taken from standard medical and scientific texts. My intention is to present the reader the opportunity to view with knowledgeable skepticism some long-held theories and to show how applications of the principles set forth here have aided the patients who have sought my assistance and followed recommendations grounded on these principles. In order to appreciate the information presented here, an open-minded ability to entertain new ideas is essential.

Whenever possible, I have based my work on established references. However, references have not always been available to substantiate the results of my research. When confronted with this situation, I try to determine what would be natural and proceed from that vantage point.

FOURTH ASSUMPTION: THERE ARE ONLY THREE CAUSES OF ILLNESS — TOXICITY, TIMING AND THOUGHTS

My experience and research have brought me to the fourth assumption (a concept introduced in Chapter One) — there are only three reasons why people are sick: Toxicity, Timing, and Thoughts.

Toxicity

Toxicity, or autointoxication, is brought about primarily by the effect on cellular metabolism of the food we eat. As we shall see, the long-term consequences of toxicity are manifest in any of an assortment of diseases, but these consequences can generally be reversed or eliminated by attention to diet, improved internal communication, and restructured thoughts.

Although toxicity is the focus of this study, timing and thoughts play far greater roles in determining our physical condition. However, as a society, we are conditioned to place more stock in quantifiable information than in the metaphysical or intangible. Consequently, while this book deals primarily with physical manifestations — toxicity — and how you, the doctor, can guide your patients on a course that will help them to allow their health to improve, a synopsis of the concepts of timing and thoughts will be helpful.

Timing

We have used the example of the stomach producing hydrochloric acid at the wrong time to illustrate a timing problem. Other areas of the body can also be affected when there is a breakdown in the body's internal communication. When a person jogs, his heart rate may increase to 120 beats per minute or more — a perfectly normal response of the body to the stress of physical exertion. When the jogger stops running and sits down to rest, his heart rate should return to normal in a matter of a few minutes. If the heart rate does not slow to a normal rate within a short period of time, a timing problem exists; the body is exhibiting a perfect response to stress, but that stress no longer exists.

Improper timing can also create new or affect existing musculoskeletal problems. It is quite common for a person who is involved in a rear-end automobile accident to sustain a whiplash injury. His entire neck and shoulder area tightens up and the range of motion of the neck is severely restricted. This is a normal reaction to an accident of this type since ligaments and muscles have reacted to a violent, traumatic situation. Normal healing of such an injury should occur within a few weeks. However, if six weeks have passed and the person is still experiencing neck stiffness, pain, and restricted motion, a timing problem exists. These conditions are normal responses to the type of trauma involved but they are not normal six weeks later. The neck and shoulder muscles are still prepared to react in a way that would prevent further injury should the stimulus (accident) be repeated; they have not received the stimulus that brings about a response of relaxation.

The body is designed to react to stress. It does this continually by a variety of means ranging from a slight altering of body temperature to reducing the blood supply to the area of an open wound. The adrenal glands (located atop each kidney) are the organs designed to deal initially with stress by producing adrenalin (dopamine, norepinephrine, and epinephrine). Adrenalin causes some body functions to speed up while others are slowed in order to respond to an emergency situation, either real or imagined. Each cell that is called upon to respond functions at a slightly faster rate which, in turn, produces more acid. These reactions to stress are normal and are designed to be short-lived — to take care of the emergency — then to return to natural function. When the doctor encounters a patient who has responded physiologically to a stressful situation and the situation has been resolved but the patient's body is still responding to it, the patient very likely is suffering from a timing problem.

Thoughts

As a doctor, your treatments already produce a certain level of positive results. My experience has shown that if you are able to motivate your patients to alter their diets to include more health-restoring, health-maintaining foods, your patient-improvement rate will rise. Ultimately, it is the patient who needs to understand and accept the fact that his symptoms are the result of his life style; his life style is the result of his habits; his habits are the result of his preferences; and his preferences are a direct result of his beliefs. If the patient is not content to accept the particular disease that is the result of his life style, habits, and preferences, he must change his beliefs.

To change a long-established belief, a person must first acknowledge that he has reached a turning point in his life that requires that he accept a new idea — a new direction in which to move. He must be committed to the idea. To fulfill the commitment, the person needs to have this idea in mind often and, most important, the idea needs to be reinforced by a deep and powerful emotion. With an amalgamation of the idea and the emotions, the cortex is occupied with the new positive idea and draws its attention away from the former habit-entrenched negative idea.

Most New Year's resolutions fail because of a lack of commitment. The person may recognize that something in his life style is contrary to a long- and deeply-held conviction and he may determine to change his ways. However, without the repetitive reinforcement of strong feelings connected with the idea, it will not take root and grow. The person will merely be doing something that he *thinks* rationally he "should" do — not something that he *feels* sensorially he "will" do. The difference between "should" and "will" is commitment.

The body does not make a decision whether or not to respond to stress. It will respond. And the response is the same whether the stress is real or imagined. Stress that is brought about by our thoughts is equally as stimulating to physiology as is stress brought about by an actual event — reality is in the perception of the individual, and the body responds with the same intensity to perceived danger as it does to actual physical danger. We have all experienced a surge of alarm brought about by anticipating a crisis — the telephone ringing in the middle of the night, or a loved one being overly late in returning from a trip — only to find that our misgivings were unwarranted. However, as far as the body is concerned, the crisis was very real.

Anxiety is an example of imaginary — or thought induced — stress. Anxiety is man-made stress — self-induced stress. Fear, anger, hate, envy, and guilt are all self-inflicted stresses that the body responds to in exactly the same way as it does to a substantive threat or situation. Adrenalin is secreted and cellular metabolism is accelerated which leads to additional acid production. But anxiety is not short-lived. It is continual — unremitting stress that signals the body to be "on guard" and ready for fight or flight. Cellular metabolism remains in a constant high speed state, producing more and more acid which, as we shall discuss in subsequent chapters, even the best diet is unable to neutralize.

Toxicity, timing and thoughts are intricately related. Each of these manifestations is present, to some degree, in each patient. The vegetarian who is extraordinarily food conscious may be plagued by negative thoughts or anxiety that speed metabolism within the cells and produce more acid. An extremely toxic patient may be extremely negative and pessimistic and suffer from "acid indigestion." Only by addressing each area — Toxicity, Timing, and Thoughts — can the patient achieve total health. Although most patients are looking for overt treatment of their physical symptoms, they can accept the importance of adjusting their diets if evidence of improved health comes not only in the form of feeling better but also of seeing better clinical test results.

EVALUATING HEALTH

Although the body is perfect in design, it will eventually suffer from prolonged abuse or neglect. To help patients improve their overall health, doctors need to be able to accurately assess the patient's degree of well-being. A major tool for this assessment is urinalysis.

The urinalysis should be considered as a monitoring device as well as an evaluation aid. In fact, I believe that a thorough urinalysis, complete with an indican test, is the easiest, least expensive and most accurate health monitor available. I believe that it is the responsibility of any doctor to be able to tell a patient just how well that patient is — where he stands on a health scale of 1 to 10. By understanding, correlating, and monitoring the results of urinalysis, the doctor can gain some of the most accurate information available to determine not only how healthy a person is but also the measures required for improvement.

Although modern medicine is 90% testing and 10% treatment, physicians still cannot give a reasonably good estimate of a patient's overall health quotient. For example, an electrocardiogram (EKG) is an excellent device that will indicate the extent of cardiac damage inflicted by a heart attack, but it cannot assess the health of the patient. Unfortunately, it is not particularly uncommon to hear of an asymptomatic individual who died of a heart attack only an hour or so after having recorded a perfect EKG. Urinalysis, on the other hand, won't tell you the extent of damage to a heart, but it will tell you the patient's level of health, and it poses no threat.

Careful monitoring of urine pH and an understanding of the ramifications of acid/alkaline imbalance are invaluable in guiding patients to health. The objective is to promote maximum healing by reducing the toxicity of the patient while monitoring his urine pH during cleansing to assure that the process is not so rapid that colds or bladder infections develop. If detoxification, or cleansing, takes place too rapidly, the patient will experience unpleasant symptoms, become discouraged, and revert to his old habits. This reversion may alleviate the symptoms but will do nothing to stem the tide of deteriorating health. The patient must be kept on a healing level which allows him to feel as good as possible during the transition period. Everyone gets well at his own pace, and the doctor needs to be aware of each individual's pace in order to be of maximum help. Monitoring urine and saliva pH can provide this information.

Saliva pH readings are equally as important as urine pH readings in determining a patient's acid/alkaline balance. Saliva pH will generally follow the pattern of the urine pH; as the urine pH rises, the saliva pH also rises but at a much slower rate. Often when a patient shows a very alkaline urine, the saliva will register acid. If the patient is on a high-protein diet, this high/low combination is an indication that the kidneys can no longer reabsorb vitally needed minerals. Consequently, a high urine pH with a low saliva reading indicates that the buffers are becoming progressively less capable of functioning as designed. Cases such as this illustrate how urinalysis results can cause confusion. Without being aware of the patient's eating habits and other personal information, the conclusions drawn from the urinalysis could be completely wrong. Keep in mind that a person is a total entity and that nothing happens in isolation. Every stimulus, either internal or external, elicits a response and every response or activity is the result of at least two stimuli — one that alerts the body to the need for action or response and one that initiates the action or response itself.

Comprehensive monitoring of urine pH and saliva pH can provide a road map to lasting health. The body must rid itself of materials that interfere with normal metabolism. These materials often show up in urine. The information provided by urinalysis can help us to reach our goal of achieving normalization of the whole body that will provide our patients the greatest level of health no matter what medical diagnostic term is used to identify a malfunction. An attempt at a quick cure, if at all successful, will merely result in the suppression of symptoms.

LOOKING AHEAD

With the four underlying assumptions in place and a brief look at how monitoring urine pH and saliva pH can aid in assessing the progress of patients, the chapters that follow deal with various aspects of physiological and biochemical reactions of the body to diet and lifestyle. You will learn why apparently healthful activities, such as jogging, can cause serious disease, and how the nutritional practices of seemingly healthy people are leading them on an unswerving path to chronic degenerative disease. And, of course, you will learn how to read the signs indicating that these conditions are present, and you will become aware of the measures that can be taken to halt or reverse the course of disease.

In this book we will describe several ways to evaluate and monitor health, and we urge you to use them all. However, I am not advocating a strictly laboratory analysis of health — my goal is for everyone who reads this book to become more aware of what the body is saying. Learn to communicate with the body — listen to it. Our bodies continually give us information not only through aches and pains but through more subtle means. Our moods, outlook, appreciation, the way we sleep, our energy level and elimination all provide bits of information that need to be considered and noted. Heeding our body's signals and communication will tell us what we need to do, what to eat, when to rest, when to drink — all of the things that the body needs to do in order to function properly.

3

IMPLICATIONS OF pH IN URINALYSIS

A REVIEW OF THE POTENTIAL OF HYDROGEN (pH)

During my investigations into nutrition and diet and their influence on our general health, the subject of pH kept reappearing. I studied protein and ran into pH; the relationships of enzymes inevitably lead to pH; urine, blood, liver — pH and its influence relates critically to each of these areas. No other single indicator is encountered as often in assessing health and disease.

The potential of Hydrogen, referred to as pH, is a measurement of the relative acidity or alkalinity of a solution. It is a scale, like a yardstick or a thermometer. The reference point for the temperature at which water freezes is 32° on a Fahrenheit thermometer; the neutral reference point on the pH scale is 7.0 indicating that a solution is neither acid nor alkaline. A pH of 8 is slightly alkaline while a pH of 12 is very alkaline; a pH of 6 is slightly acid, and a pH of 3 is very acid.

Hydrogen ions make a solution acid, and the pH value indicates the number of additional hydrogen ions a solution has the potential of holding or accepting. Since the pH scale is structured in inverse order, the more hydrogen ions present, the lower the pH number. As a simple example, at pH 9, only five hydrogen ions are present and the solution is quite alkaline. At pH 2, there are already twelve hydrogen ions present, making the solution highly acid. When the number is below 7.0, an acid state exists. The fewer hydrogen ions present, the higher the pH number and the more alkaline the solution. Or, to put it another way, the pH number reflects inversely the number of hydrogen ions present — or, the ability (or potential) of the solution to gain more hydrogen ions.

Recall that in physiological oxidation the removal of hydrogen ions or electrons is involved. As these hydrogen ions are taken from one substance and attached to another, the pH changes and the relative acid-alkaline balance changes.

pH Scale of Acidic Reaction

	A C I D			NEUTRAL	A L K A L I N E			
Total	Very	Moderate	Slight		Slight	Moderate	Very	Total
0 1	2	3 4	5 6	7	8 9	10 11	12 13	14

Keep in mind that the pH scale represents a logarithm which means that the difference between each unit is tenfold; pH 5 is ten times more acid than pH 6 while pH 4 is one hundred times more acid than pH 6.

It is interesting and important to note that in the body only the stomach fluids are inherently acid. All of the body's systems should be alkaline — blood, interstitial fluid, lymph, intracellular fluid, extracellular fluid, cerebrospinal fluid are alkaline — only the stomach fluids should be acid.

The human body is an acid producing organism by function, yet it is an alkaline organism by design. Acid is produced in the stomach by the parietal cells of the gastric mucousa to aid in the digestion of food. However, we find no cells that similarly produce alkali. Where, then, does the alkalinity come from? To answer this question as well as to grasp the relationship of pH to health and to correlate this with the role nutrition plays in this relationship, it is necessary to understand the effects that acid, as indicated by pH levels, have on the many organs and systems of the body.

pH, HEALTH, AND RESEARCH

Most authors and researchers who have delved into an investigation of pH have recognized the vital role it plays in our overall health. Yet, whether the researcher is a medical doctor, chiropractor, or Ph.D., the true relationship between pH and good health has consistently been missed. Research has followed the pH chain back through the digestive process without connecting the final link. Some researchers have come so close that their recommendations are correct — but their reasons are wrong.

In *The 2nd Factor in Chiropractic*, the paradox of acidifying foods producing an apparent alkaline condition is described.

> "If overcoming an alkalinity were it as simple as the correction of an acidity, there would be no problem at all. In correcting an acidity we need only to have patients eat alkalizing foods, the various fruits, or eat the neutralizing foods, the leafy vegetables. But with an alkalinity it is different. *People become too alkaline — strange as it may appear — by eating acidizing foods.* Therefore giving patients more of such foods would only worsen their conditions."[1] [Emphasis added]

To add to the confusion and misconceptions concerning alkalinity, most patients who experience bladder infections have an alkaline urine, but not all patients with an alkaline urine experience bladder infections.

A first-hand experience illustrated how an alkaline urine reading can lead to a misdiagnosis if the origin of the alkalinity is not understood.

When I was in the hospital for treatment of a broken hip caused by an automobile accident, I did not eat the food served by the hospital. I didn't know as much about nutrition then as I do now, but I did know that my body needed fruits and vegetables for maximum healing, so I had my family bring me carrot juice and fresh peach juice. When urinalysis revealed about 8.0 pH, the doctors, who apparently equated alkaline urine with major pathological conditions, wanted to put me on antibiotics immediately. I suggested that they culture the urine to isolate the offending bacteria, and of course, the culture revealed no bacteria. This situation was very confusing to physicians who were not accustomed to seeing a decidedly alkaline urine in the absence of infection. They had not recognized the link between acidosis that masquerades as alkalinity and the depletion of the alkaline reserve.

Guyton uses a very complex formula to determine pH from the ratio of carbonic acid to bicarbonate.[2] He indicates that the alkaline reserve is simply the ability of bicarbonate ions to combine with a mineral (sodium) to form a salt which the body can eliminate. Apparently, he assumes that everyone has an adequate supply of sodium available from the sodium chloride (table salt) that is eaten with meals. He seems to have completely missed the critical point that without adequate organic sodium derived from fruits and vegetables, the bicarbonate ions will have nothing with which to combine and, therefore, no acid-buffering salt will be formed. The body cannot use either the sodium or the chlorine from table salt since these elements are held together tightly by ionic bonds. The body is designed to utilize substances that are covalently bonded — that is, substances that are joined by bonds that are easily broken and rearranged. Only covalently bonded organic sodium is usable by the body and its buffering systems.

Royal Lee (who is well known throughout the chiropractic profession) made a similar mistake in equating electrovalent minerals with covalent minerals when he used Cal-Amo and Phosfood to relieve bladder irritation. Both of these substances are totally inorganic; they have no physiological function at all as far as nutrition is concerned. But they do have a palliative effect if the patient has eaten too much meat. These substances will immediately return the urine to an acid condition even though there is an excess of ammonia and bicarbonate. The entire urinary tract is then acidified and the patient feels better. Distilled apple cider vinegar would accomplish the same thing since all of the alkalizing agents are removed in the distillation process of the apple juice leaving only pure acetic acid. "Distilled" apple cider vinegar is recommended only for the patient who is experiencing bladder irritation and whose urinalysis confirms excess ammonia.

pH AND CELLS

As we have stated, the stomach is naturally acid. The parietal (or oxyntic) cells of the gastric glands produce hydrochloric acid (HCl) as a part of the digestive process. Although we consume acid (in fruits such as lemons), produce acid (lactic acid generated by muscle activity), and eliminate acid (uric acid from the kidneys), we should remain an alkaline organism overall.

The table below shows the pH ranges that are considered medically normal to specific body substances and areas.

pH Table[3,4,5]

Blood	7.35 - 7.45
Saliva	6.50 - 7.50
Gastric	1.00 - 3.50
Duodenum	4.80 - 8.20
Feces	4.60 - 8.40
Urine	4.50 - 8.40
Liver Bile	7.10 - 8.50
Gall Bladder Bile	5.50 - 7.70
Pancreas	8.00 - 8.30

In recognizing the delicate nature of systemic pH balance, Guyton states: "Only slight changes in hydrogen ion concentration from the normal value cause marked alterations in the rates of chemical reactions in the cells, some being depressed and others accelerated."[6]

The intracellular chemical reactions to which Guyton refers are very specialized and critical. The body lives or dies at the cellular level and all cellular functions are controlled by enzymes. It follows that if pH affects enzymes, it will also affect the function of the cells. We are familiar with the digestive enzymes ptyalin, lipase, amylase, and pepsin and we recognize them as complex proteins that can alter other substances without being changed themselves. However, the digestive enzymes are but a small segment of the complex enzyme spectrum. Many very specialized enzymes function inside each cell guiding its structure and function; any alteration in the pH inside or around the cell can have far-reaching consequences. Therefore, maintaining optimum pH is paramount to maintaining optimum health. If the cells are healthy, the person is healthy; if the cells cannot function properly, the person becomes sick; if sufficient numbers of cells die, the person dies.

Every cell utilizes glucose for energy; whether it is a brain cell or a bone cell, the intrinsic function is much the same and the cell requires glucose for fuel. Glucose is transferred through the cell wall by insulin. The optimum pH in which the hormone insulin functions is 7.8 to 8.0. Since moving glucose through the cell wall is the main function of insulin and since insulin functions most efficiently at a pH of 7.8 to 8.0, all extracellular fluids should be within this pH range. If the pH varies from this range, some cellular function will be depressed or accelerated thereby affecting total body physiology.[7]

OXIDATION AND ENERGY

Every school child is taught that oxygen is carried to the cells by the blood. The amount of oxygen available in the blood determines how efficiently oxidation will occur within the cells. Oxidation is the process of combining a substance with oxygen to produce heat or energy. An illustration of oxidation is seen when an apple is cut and the inside immediately begins to turn brown; the apple is oxidizing. This type of oxidation should take place inside the body to produce energy. Physiological oxidation usually does not involve the addition of oxygen at high temperatures but involves the removal of hydrogen or simply the removal of electrons.

Glucose is combined with oxygen in the mitochondria of the cells to produce adenosine triphosphate (ATP) which provides high energy bonds that supply the body with energy. ATP production can occur without oxygen. However, when cells make ATP without oxygen (anaerobic glycolysis) only 3 molecules of ATP per mol of glucose are produced as opposed to between 32 and 36 molecules of ATP per glucose mol when sufficient oxygen is present — ample oxygen yields a tenfold difference in ATP production.[8] Research indicates that blood carries the maximum amount of oxygen to the cells at the specific pH of 7.4.[9]

Since (1) the amount of oxygen available determines the type of oxidation that occurs within the cells, and (2) blood pH must be between 7.35 and 7.45, and (3) the point at which the blood will carry the maximum amount of oxygen is 7.4 pH, it then follows that both blood and interstitial fluid need to be alkaline in order for cells to function maximally.

BUFFERS THAT MAINTAIN HOMEOSTASIS

The body is designed to maintain the pH levels that are vitally necessary to survival; several methods exist for keeping acid/base balances within acceptable limits. Three main control systems act in harmony to maintain the required balance: 1) kidneys, 2) lungs, and 3) buffer systems. The kidneys have the ability to excrete either an acid or alkaline urine; the lungs can change their rate of respiration thereby altering the carbon dioxide concentration and pH; and the intricate bicarbonate, phosphate, and protein buffer systems can alter the pH of all body fluids.

A buffer is a substance that preserves the original hydrogen-ion concentration of a solution when either an acid or base is added. It is made up of an acid and a base. For example, the bicarbonate buffer has both carbonic acid and bicarbonate present. Guyton indicates that the bicarbonate buffer is made up of approximately 20 times more bicarbonate ions than dissolved carbon dioxide, giving it a ratio of 20:1.[10] If an acid is added, the substance will become more acid; if an alkali is added, the substance will become more alkaline. The point at which the buffering systems come into balance or equilibrium (the ionization constant of a buffer solution) is called pK. The closer the pH of a system is to the pK of that system, the greater the buffering power.

The body's different systems for maintaining the acid-alkaline balance work at vastly differing speeds within various pH ranges. Although the lungs can effectively begin to eliminate acid in minutes and can eliminate one hundred times more acid than can other systems, they are a relatively weak pH-maintaining system. The kidneys are a strong system but require from five hours to several days to eliminate the acid of body metabolism. On the other hand, the buffers can respond in seconds. Each of these systems is designed to cover a specific area of acid-alkaline balance, yet, all work together in harmony. Guyton points out the importance of the isohydric principle that can affect the workings of each of the buffer systems. ". . . any condition that changes the balance of any one of the buffer systems also changes the balance of all the others, for *the buffer systems actually buffer each other by shifting hydrogen ions from one to the other.*"[11]

Not only do the three buffer systems (bicarbonate, phosphate, and protein) react at different speeds and overlap activities, they also cover different pH ranges. The interrelation of the three systems can be compared to a three-speed manual automobile transmission. We start out in low gear with the bicarbonate buffer taking the pH to 6.1. We then shift into second, the phosphate buffer, to advance the pH to 6.8. Finally, we get up to speed in third gear with the protein buffer at 7.4. To carry the analogy of the automobile transmission one step further, we do most of our driving in third gear just as most of the buffering in the body is done by the protein buffer system. However, if we want to reach a speed of 55 MPH, we must first go through the lower gears. Similarly, the three buffer systems are called upon to respond to a variety of imbalances in different systems in the body.

BICARBONATE BUFFER SYSTEM

The bicarbonate buffer system is the first equilibrium-maintaining system to respond to a change in the acid/alkaline balance. This system operates extracellularly and is important in regulating blood and interstitial fluid pH. When protein (either animal or vegetable) digestion produces an acid, such as sulfuric, that has a pH of less than 6.1, the bicarbonate buffer can react in seconds. This is not a particularly powerful system but it is easily regulated by the body. The pK of the bicarbonate buffer system is 6.1 and we have seen that the pH of the blood should be maintained at 7.4. The bicarbonate buffer falls far short of reaching the degree of alkalinity the blood requires, but it is an important first step.

Sodium and other alkaline reserve minerals are vital to the functioning of this buffer since they combine with bicarbonate ions to form sodium bicarbonate and other acid salts that accomplish the buffering process. The acid salts are eliminated in the urine. This buffering process is so effective that the blood can take three hundred times more acid than can an equal volume of water before the same change in pH is reached.[12] However, when this process takes place in the body, sodium is lost in the urine.

PHOSPHATE BUFFER SYSTEM

The phosphate buffer system, although similar to the bicarbonate buffer, differs in that it functions primarily inside the cell using potassium rather than sodium as the buffer. Phosphate is much more heavily concentrated inside the cell than outside. Although this system can operate in extracellular fluid, its buffering capabilities outside the cell are minimal. The phosphate buffer system operates efficiently inside the cell since intracellular pH is much closer than extracellular pH to 6.8 pK of the phosphate buffer system.

Essentially, the phosphate buffer acts to change strong acid to weak acid. Potassium, as found in usable covalent form in fruits and vegetables, is essential for the proper functioning of the phosphate buffer which is designed to bring the pH of the cell to approximately 6.8. If adequate amounts of fruits and vegetables are not consumed, the amount of potassium inside the cell decreases and the phosphate buffer system will not function properly.

PROTEIN BUFFER SYSTEM

The third and most powerful of the buffering systems, the protein buffer system, further fine-tunes pH.

The proteins referred to here are protein molecules that have been absorbed and function within the cells where approximately 75% of all buffering takes place. The pK of this system is 7.4 — the desired pH of blood. Proteins are composed of amino acids, many of which can easily accept or reject a hydrogen ion. The protein molecule is a living structure — it is not static. Protein is dynamic — constantly twisting and turning. It has the ability to change its configuration by twisting and taking off a hydrogen or hydroxal and connecting two elements together.

Protein buffers in and of itself. A protein that is complete and intact will do its buffering by changing its configuration. Phosphate and bicarbonate must combine or join with a "partner" such as potassium, sodium, or calcium in order to accomplish the buffering, and as a result, these elements are lost in the urine.

It may appear inconsistent to say that 75% of all buffering is accomplished intracellularly by the protein buffer system and, at the same time, claim that large amounts of protein are harmful. There is no inconsistency since two separate situations are involved.

First, the protein buffer system is effective only in the limited pH range between 6.8 to 7.4; it is not capable of changing a pH of 5.5 to 7.4.

None of the buffer systems work independently — their processes overlap to some degree. For example, imagine that the body has been engaged in physical activity and lactic acid has been produced by the muscles during exercise. After a period of rest, the body should return to intracellular and extracellular equalization at a minimum of pH 6.1 which is the pK of the lowest buffer system — the bicarbonate system. After an interval of time and rest, equilibrium should reach 6.8, the pK of the phosphate buffer system; and with complete rest it should rise to 7.4, the pK of the protein buffer system. However, the initial 25% of the buffering process must be accomplished by the bicarbonate and phosphate systems before the 75% of the process performed by the protein system can be effective.

Excess protein causes more acid to be formed in the cells, and over time, sodium for buffering is depleted and the phosphate inside the cells is "handicapped" by excess protein. However, a small amount of protein inside the cells cannot effectively buffer the additional load so the cells take on excessive amounts of protein. The result is that the protein within the cells is required to take on a bigger role in the buffering process.

Second, we are referring to excess protein being harmful — more protein than the cells need or can use effectively. Although every cell must contain protein, and cells need protein in the buffering process, excess protein inside the cells interferes with normal function.

Protein is necessary to maintain life. But, as we shall see, when we consistently consume excessive amounts of protein, vital supplies of sodium and potassium are exhausted, and the bicarbonate and phosphate buffer systems are unable to function. The cells then try to use intracellular protein to compensate for the lack of the first two buffer systems.

Excess protein inside the cells becomes pathological in an attempt to perform physiological functions. Since protein is a buffer and works as a buffer, as the body becomes more acid, more protein is necessary to neutralize the acidity. More protein is then taken into the cells to perform the buffering and even though the desired 7.4 pH may be reached, the excess protein causes further cell congestion and deterioration.

When the cell is congested with protein, it cannot function properly. More water is then taken into the cell to dilute the protein and preserve the osmotic balance. This allows the cell to function in as nearly normal fashion as possible under the circumstances.

Every chemical reaction in the human body takes place in a water medium. Cells use $C_6H_{12}O_6$ (glucose) for ATP production in a water medium. Hydrogen is removed from glucose enzymatically and combines with the O_2 of air to make H_2O which can be eliminated by the kidneys. Also, CO_2 is produced in the cell through Krebs cycle. With the enzyme carbonic anhydrase in every cell acting as a catalyst, the CO_2 combines with H_2O to form H_2CO_3 (carbonic acid). Some of this is transported to the lungs where the carbonic anhydrase acts to reverse the process thereby forming CO_2 and H_2O. Some of the CO_2 and water vapor can be exhaled. The rest of the water can be eliminated through the kidneys.

Excess water in the cells as a result of excess protein in the diet contributes to a condition commonly referred to as edema or dropsy — not Natural, nor Normal, but certainly Necessary. The key is that excess protein sets in motion a series of reactions that require protein to try to buffer more than it was designed to handle.

As a result, we have a "catch-22" situation. Additional protein causes additional acid which must be neutralized. The increased buffering requirements can reduce the efficiency of the bicarbonate and phosphate buffer systems so the protein buffer system moves into high gear which, in turn, generates more acid which requires more protein. As this cycle is perpetuated, it culminates in the development of chronic degenerative disease, and drugs may be used to eliminate the water from the body.

SUMMARY

The body functions under the conditions inflicted upon it, and the food consumed produces these conditions. By monitoring a patient's pH, an accurate picture of his health is available. When pH varies radically from the system's or organ's pK, the patient is not in the optimum state of health and sensitive systems and organs must function under adverse circumstances. This combination of conditions will ultimately lead to chronic degenerative disease — arthritis, diabetes, and osteoporosis, to name a few.

Excessive amounts of protein in any form, whether animal protein or the protein of legumes and other plant foods, is debilitating to the body. Protein is essential to good health, but excess protein assures that poor health is inevitable. The addition of fruits and vegetables to the patient's diet will provide the vitamins, minerals, and complete protein required to keep the body functioning, comfortable, and healthy. Monitoring pH is the most accurate method of determining a patient's progress and overall level of health.

If the patient who is normally on a high-protein diet begins to eat large quantities of fruits and vegetables, his urine may register alkaline and he may develop a bladder infection. If he then eats more protein he will feel better since the protein may return the urine pH to the acidity his body is accustomed to. The problem is that the kidneys are already overtaxed and the additional protein simply adds to the overload. A better way to re-acidify is with cranberry juice, or distilled vinegar, which will neutralize excess ammonia. For all other uses — medicinal and as ingredients in culinary preparations such as salad dressing — only pure *non-distilled* apple cider vinegar that has the alkalizing agents intact is recommended.

The urine of a patient who regularly eats high-protein foods can be alkaline. When excess protein is consumed, ammonia is eliminated in the urine and bicarbonate will be in the urine as a result of the stomach producing hydrochloric acid to digest the protein. Normally the bicarbonate would attach to a sodium ion to form sodium bicarbonate, but when the sodium has been depleted, the bicarbonate is not reabsorbed and is lost in the urine. These two factors give a misleading alkaline urine pH readings. If the urine is alkaline due to excess protein consumption, the more protein consumed, the more alkaline the urine becomes. By understanding this process, we can answer the question posed at the beginning of this book, "How can eating acidifying foods, such as animal protein, result in an increasingly alkaline urine?"

4

METABOLIC ASH AND THE EFFECTS OF FOOD

ACID ASH AND ALKALINE ASH

The concept of "acid-ash-producing" foods and "alkaline-ash-producing" foods as referred to in this study may not be clearly understood by some patients. These terms apply to the ASH of food that remains after the nutrients have been removed in the digestive process, not necessarily to the food itself. To clarify this concept, we can offer a simplified review of the digestive process.

The alimentary canal can be thought of as being external to the body — similar to the hole in a doughnut. Food goes into the mouth and is processed in the stomach. Some of the properties of the food are absorbed in the small intestine and the remainder goes into the large intestine, eventually to be eliminated in the stool. The part that was not absorbed never actually "entered" the body — it had no role in nourishing the body and serves only as bulk in the large intestine.

The portion of the food that actually became a part of the body was absorbed, usually through the small intestine. This fraction of the food is metabolized and utilized by the body.

Following metabolism, any portion of this small fraction that is "left over," or not utilized, is termed "ash." Some of this ash is acid in nature, some is alkaline; however, **the acidity or alkalinity of the ash is not necessarily the same as that of the food in its original state before being eaten.**

For example, a lemon has a pH of approximately 2.5 or 3.0; it is highly acid. Parts of the lemon that are fiber and other substances not absorbed by the body pass through the digestive tract to be eliminated in the stool. The part of the highly acid lemon that is absorbed and metabolized yields a highly alkaline ash of about pH 9. A soda cracker, on the other hand, is neutral in its original state but the remaining ash is very acid. There is a clear distinction between "ash," the retained portion of metabolized food, and digestive "residue," the portion of food neither absorbed nor metabolized that passes directly through the body.

Ash results from the digestion of both animal and vegetable foods. The ash that remains after digestion of animal protein, dairy products, eggs, and grains is acid, while the ash of most fruit and vegetable digestion is generally alkaline. Foods such as syrups, fats, oils, white sugar and other processed or synthetic foods leave no ash but have an acidifying effect on the body. They are high-energy foods that force the body to metabolize glucose rapidly which causes the cells to produce more acid. However, the acid produced is carbonic acid (H_2CO_3) that can be eliminated through the lungs. When additional acid, even carbonic acid that can be exhaled or lactic acid produced by exercise, is generated in a body that is already heavily acid, the results can be serious.

The critical difference between the foods of the Standard American Diet and junk food diet is the type and amount of residual ash the body must process. Digestion of the high-protein steak-and-eggs diet produces strong inorganic acids, such as nitric and sulfuric, that must be neutralized before they can be eliminated in the urine. Junk food is principally highly refined carbohydrates that yield smaller quantities of inorganic acid ash and take less of the alkaline reserve to neutralize. Although neither of these diets contributes adequate amounts of minerals to the alkaline reserve, the rate at which the junk food diet depletes the reserve is slower than that of the high-protein Standard American Diet.

Acid ash and alkaline ash are pivotal factors of health. How ash affects metabolism, homeostasis, and the general well-being of the body is an underlying theme of both good health and this book. When patients (and doctors) know which foods leave the type of ash the body can eliminate with the least amount of stress, and which foods produce the most un-favorable conditions for the body, they can control their diets so that the body can function optimally.

The following lists show in descending order of potency some of the most common foods in the alkaline-ash producing and acid-ash producing categories.

ALKALINE ASH FOODS	ACID ASH FOODS
Raw spinach	Scallops
Beet greens	Oysters
Molasses	Dried lentils
Celery	Sausage
Dried figs	Sardines
Carrots	Oatmeal
Dried beans	Corned beef
Chard leaves	Lobster
Watercress	Peanuts
Sauerkraut	Haddock
Lettuce	Soda crackers
Green Lima beans	Codfish
Dried Lima beans	Macaroni, Spaghetti
*Rhubarb	Peanut butter
Cabbage	Chicken
Broccoli	Pike
Beets	Wheat germ
Brussels sprouts	Brown rice
Green soy beans	Whole wheat flour
Cucumbers	White flour
Parsnips	Salmon
Radishes	Beef
Rutabagas	Turkey

(DIMINISHING ALKALINE ASH — DIMINISHING ACID ASH)

ALKALINE ASH FOODS	ACID ASH FOODS
Dried peas	Barley
Mushrooms	Veal
Cauliflower	Lamb
Pineapple	White bread
Avocado	Wheat bran
Raisins	English walnuts
Dried dates	Bacon
Green beans	Eggs
Muskmelon	Whole wheat bread
Limes	Pork
Sour cherries	Honey
Tangerines	Shrimp
Strawberries	Fresh corn
White potatoes	
Sweet potatoes	
Grapefruit	
Apricots	
Lemons	
Blackberries	NEUTRAL ASH WITH
Oranges	ACIDIFYING EFFECT
Tomatos	
Peaches	Refined sugar
Raspberries	Corn oil
Bananas	Olive oil
Onions	Corn syrup
Grapes	
Pears	
Blueberries	
Apples	
Watermelon	
Green Peas	
* Not Recommended	

As this list illustrates, alkaline-ash producing foods come, essentially, from the plant kingdom — fruits and vegetables. Acid-ash producing foods are generally protein and refined carbohydrates.

The concept of acid ash/alkaline ash is vital to this study of urinalysis and much of the information in this section will be elaborated in other chapters. The reader should keep in mind that the term "excess protein" refers to that amount of protein over and above the amounts the human body can process efficiently and use beneficially to support bodily functions. Excess protein creates large amounts of acid. It is important to keep in mind that the body must deal with the chemical properties of this acid in the best way it can. A brief overview concerning the bonding of chemical substances may be helpful.

CHEMICAL BONDS AND NEUTRALIZING MINERALS

A chemical bond is the linkage between different atoms or radicals of a chemical compound. Some of these bonds are extremely strong, others are quite weak. All chemical reaction requires a replacement involvement — exchange will take place in a compound only if some substance or element can be replaced by something else.

Through the miracle of photosynthesis, nature combines two kingdoms: the plant kingdom and the mineral kingdom. The food we eat should come from the plant kingdom which is the only source of food in the form that the body can utilize most efficiently. We are unable to use the minerals from the mineral kingdom because of the way the atoms or ions of these elements are bonded — the way they are joined together.

In chemistry, there are two kinds of bonding: *ionic*, in which the ions or atoms are held together tightly, and *covalent*, with ions or atoms that are held together very loosely and are easily separated.

Covalent bonds can be easily separated when a pair of shared electrons spin in opposite directions between two atoms. Ionic bonds formed by electromagnetic attraction are much stronger than covalent bonds. The body's enzyme system can be used to break bonds that are formed by electrons spinning in opposite directions rather than dealing with totally electric positive or negative situations. The body is designed to work with covalent rather than with ionic bonds which is why minerals other than those found in fruits and vegetables are not easily assimilated for use by the body. There is a stronger action between positive and negative elements, such as sodium and chloride, and the attraction is so strong that the body is unable to sever the association. The body has the ability to slow down and break apart spinning electrons rather than the ability to break an electromotive attraction between two substances.

As a general rule, the elements of the mineral kingdom are held together tightly by ionic bonding while bonding of the vegetable kingdom is covalent — loosely held. The difference between the mineral kingdom and vegetable kingdom for our purposes is the type of bonding — one very strong and rigid, the other weak and loose. The human body is capable of breaking loose bonds. The air we breathe, the water we drink and all of the substances the body uses effectively are covalently bonded — but the body is unable to break the rigid ionic bonds of the mineral kingdom. For example, the bond between the sodium and chloride of table salt (NaCl) is so strong that few other substances have as great an attraction for either of the element's ions as they have for each other; consequently, no replacement occurs. Both sodium and chloride are extremely active elements — they have a great attraction for each other even after complete disassociation in water. This strong attraction prevents the body from using the sodium.

Patients should be cautioned not to confuse sodium with sodium chloride. In recent years, medical authorities have emphasized the importance of restricting salt intake. Inorganic sodium — sodium chloride — should be avoided; however, organic sodium as found in fruits and vegetables may be the most vital element in normal physiology.

Yet, analysis of blood will reveal the presence of inorganic minerals such as sodium chloride. Since salt is also found in the urine, it could be assumed that salt is being lost and that more should be consumed for replacement. However, the body is not capable of breaking the strong ionic bonds that hold the sodium and chloride together. Again we have a condition that may appear to be normal but is, in reality, necessary if the individual has eaten so much salt that the blood is the only place the body can store it. Sodium chloride has a major effect on the osmotic balance of the cells but this sodium cannot be used in the buffering process.

It takes a long time for the body to rid itself of stored salt even after table salt has been eliminated from the diet. A patient who had cancer came to me for treatment of back pain. During the first four months he came for treatment his diet consisted of nothing except raw fruit and vegetable juices. During the next two months he ate some raw fruit and vegetables and continued to drink at least a gallon of carrot juice a day. On one of his visits, he complained of having a cold; I told him that I had never known a terminal cancer patient to have a cold. In addition to the cold, he said that his lips were very dry and tasted extremely salty although he had eaten no salt for six months. He admitted to having been heavy-handed with the salt shaker before he changed his dietary habits and now, six months later, his body was still getting rid of the salt he had previously consumed.

THE EFFECT OF COOKING ON CHEMICAL BONDS

Cooking appears to alter the strength of the covalent bonds of foods. For example, as soon as milk is pasteurized, the calcium changes to a form that strongly resembles ionically bonded calcium. This calcium may appear to be in usable form and is transported through the intestinal wall into the blood stream; but the body knows the difference and "dumps" the calcium wherever it can. In the case of a 26-year old female patient who consumed large quantities of pasteurized milk, an x-ray showed definite signs of osteoporosis (which is caused by lack of calcium) along with obvious calcium deposits in the cartilage near the ribs. The body needed calcium for the bones but was putting it in places where it was not needed — the body was not in error, the calcium being deposited could not be used beneficially.

Experiments have shown that even calves will not survive on pasteurized milk. Apparently, the pasteurization process alters the milk so that it no longer meets the needs of the calf. In my opinion, this alteration has to do with the chemical bonding of the elements of pasteurized milk.

DIETS AND THE IMPACT OF CHANGE

Doctors are often surprised at how little of the food their patients eat is nutritious. Diets of cold cereal, milk and coffee for breakfast, hamburger and soft drink for lunch, and pizza for dinner are not at all uncommon — especially for younger patients. Cola drinks, the principal beverage for many Americans, are particularly detrimental to health in general and teeth in particular. Not only do they have an acidifying effect, they also contain a great deal of sugar.

However, merely encouraging patients to stop eating junk food will not influence their behavior. Motivating them through education and providing self-monitoring methods that allow them to see evidence of their state of health will help them to alter their eating habits to include the food that the body was designed to utilize. By adding beneficial foods to their daily diet rather than restricting the foods they usually eat, they will have neither the time nor the capacity to eat junk food. Anything less than total revision of eating habits is merely a half measure that will yield only temporary results.

Extreme care should be taken in altering the diet of a patient. If a person rapidly changes his diet from one that is 85% acid-ash producing to one that is 75% alkaline-ash producing he will feel worse even though his health is improving. By altering the diet gradually, adding one meal of vegetables per day and a supplement of a digestive aid enzyme with betaine hydrochloride at that meal, the body will be better able to digest the food without subjecting the patient to unpleasant physical reactions. Meat is a powerful stimulant. Few patients can be withdrawn from stimulation all at once without rather dramatic repercussions. Diet changes for patients must be gradual. As we shall see in our discussion of enzymes, their bodies have lost or modified some normal processes and must be given time to make the changes necessary to accommodate to the new diet.

Radical changes in diet can have a devastating affect on living organisms as was illustrated by a humanitarian effort that produced results diametrically opposed to those intended. A few years ago, a herd of deer was snowbound high in the mountains of Colorado. In an effort to save the deer, alfalfa hay, the same feed given to deer in zoos, was airlifted and dropped to the starving animals. Subsequent flights over the area revealed the deer had died despite the food drop, and investigations later showed that the deer had starved to death with their stomaches full of the alfalfa hay. These deer had lived in the wild on a diet of brush and tree leaves and their digestive systems could not utilize the alfalfa hay. Their enzyme systems were geared to act on the diet they had eaten all of their lives and could not adapt to the new diet in time to save them.

Enzyme production for many patients is geared to handle refined carbohydrates and will not initially be able to process such commonplace vegetables as green beans. All dietary changes must be slow enough to allow the body time to change from Necessary to Natural responses.

The effects acid-ash producing foods have on a patient can be monitored by tracking the pH levels of the saliva and urine. Even if a patient who has been accustomed to a diet high in animal protein changes his diet to include 75% vegetables and his pH levels indicate that his health is improving, his pH readings may begin to move back toward the levels he had when he was sick. In this event, he needs to increase the amount of alkaline-ash producing foods in his diet. Patients need not be concerned about "giving up meat"; if they eat enough vegetables and fruits the body will be provided with ample protein, and meat will give them up — they will lose their taste and desire for meat. It may take a year or more for this preference change to occur — but given time, it will happen.

EXPANSIVE AND CONTRACTIVE FOODS

Foods that inflict high dietary stress on the body can be described as being "expansive" or "contractive." Other foods fall into a category described as "neutral"; they impose little, if any, stress on bodily functions.

The table that follows shows general food groups in the "expansive," "neutral," and "contractive" categories. The substances named at the top and bottom of the chart represent extremes, i.e., drugs are the most expansive and salt is the most contractive, while fruit juices and butter produce the least stress of the foods in their respective groups and are very close to being neutral.

The concept that the body continuously seeks balance — homeostasis or equilibrium — is essential to understanding how contractive and expansive foods influence people's food preferences. A correlation exists between acidifying foods and contractive foods as well as between alkalizing foods and expansive foods. Contractive foods tend to restrict cells, blood vessels, and even thinking. For example, a person may eat a diet of predominantly acid-forming; contractive foods such as steak, eggs and grains but if some alkalizing foods with expansive properties, such as fruits and vegetables, are not eaten to allow the body to achieve balance, the body will seek balance through other means.

We can use the analogy of a child's seesaw to illustrate the relative impact of either adding or subtracting from the balance. If we use the center of the list — Human Milk — as the balance point and the rest of the items as positioned on either side of this point, we can see that when we remove red meat and salt from one side of the seesaw without removing counterbalancing items from the other side, a significant reaction will take place.

EXPANSIVE AND CONTRACTIVE FOODS

H I G H
S T R E S S

EXPANSIVE
Drugs — Recreational
and Prescription
Liquor
Beer
Wine
Sugar
Syrup (honey, molasses)
Chocolate
Coffee
Tea
Fruit Juice

NEUTRAL

75% Adult Diet
{ Fruits
{ Vegetables

Human Milk

25% Adult Diet
{ Grains
{ Nuts
{ Seeds
{ Beans

L O W
S T R E S S

H I G H
S T R E S S

CONTRACTIVE
Butter
Chicken
Fish
Eggs
Fowl
Red Meat
Salt

The body will achieve some measure of balance through its homeostasis-seeking tendency regardless of the food the person consumes. For example, if the person eats only contractive foods, red meat, salt, etc., and the body is not given an expansive food to balance this, the expansive balance may be achieved by sudden explosive outbursts of temper. Contractive personality traits will be exhibited if the body is denied counterbalancing expansive food. Consider this possibility in relation to the athlete who is on a high protein diet and who falls victim to recreational drug use.

On the other end of the spectrum, a strict vegetarian (whose diet consists predominantly of expansive foods) might tend to be less physically and verbally aggressive. A vegetarian may have fruit juice for breakfast, carrot juice for lunch, and a salad for dinner and become so expansive that he is unable to concentrate. He will have a thought and before he can act on it another will take its place. He will not be grounded — his mind will wander — and he will be unable to follow a thought through to completion. A patient who expresses these symptoms should eat only brown rice for two or three days. The contractive effects of the brown rice will gently and appropriately offset the expansive effects of the juices. Urine and saliva pH of the patient should be monitored carefully during this time. After a few days of the brown rice diet, the hyper-expansive patient will regain a more stable attitude and can resume eating vegetables being guided by both how he feels and urine and saliva pH readings. This is a good illustration of the body's determination to maintain balance; it reinforces the concept that each of us needs to listen to what our body is telling us. Our bodies continually give us hints that are too often ignored.

Most items shown as expansive have limited nutritional value but can be quite stimulatory. Although these foods may leave a neutral ash — neither acid nor alkaline — the ash has a decidedly acidifying effect on the body due to the rapid production of carbonic acid as the cells' mitochondria function to utilize the increased content of glucose.

In order to maintain homeostatic balance when a contractive food is eliminated from the diet, an expansive food should also be eliminated. For example, if the person is giving up red meat which is contractive, he must also give up foods that act on the body in an expansive way, such as alcohol, drugs, coffee, chocolate, and sugar.

If a patient decides to upgrade his diet and gives up only an expansive food but does not give up its counteracting contractive food, he will crave the expansive food to an extent that is almost uncontrollable and will probably gorge himself on the very food he is trying to avoid. Keep in mind that the body works toward homeostatic balance. When a certain food that is contractive is eaten, the body will crave one that is expansive in an effort to maintain balance. Craving a particular food or beverage is a clear indication that this substance, along with the food that "balances" it, should be eliminated from the diet.

VEGETARIANISM

While I strongly recommend a predominantly vegetable diet, I recognize that some vegetarians are ill. Generally, one of three factors accounts for this.

First, the body's immediate response to a rapid radical change in diet may not be favorable. It takes time for the body to begin producing the enzymes necessary to process larger quantities of fruits and vegetables. The patient can experience unpleasant repercussions from a quick change in diet — cold- or flu-like symptoms are signals that cleansing of the body is taking place too rapidly.

Second, illness of a vegetarian may be a function of the kind of vegetarian he is. Vegetarians vary in their degree of dedication to adhering strictly to plant life foods. Dairy products and/or significant quantities of grains can produce very acid ash that cannot be counteracted by the vegetables eaten. Anyone who eats more than 47 grams of protein a day — no matter what the source of the protein — will eventually develop osteoporosis.

The third factor is that although nutrition plays a major role, it is only a part of the total health picture. Interference from other sources, including attitudes and physiological timing can affect total body function.

Vegetarians are not immune to harboring negative thoughts; neither are they immune to producing acid as a consequence of negative attitudes and thoughts. We must recognize that the mind is the most powerful agent that influences physiology. A vegetarian's body may be seriously out of balance thus hindering proper timing, correct digestion, and assimilation of even healthful food. Health is a matter of correct timing, correct thoughts, and corrected toxicity.

I want to emphasize that it is not necessary for a person to become a strict vegetarian in order to be healthy. The ideal dietary ratio should be approximately 75% fruits and vegetables to 25% protein. Thirty percent of the fruits and vegetables should be eaten raw, and the protein should come from grains, seeds, nuts, and, if desired, meat, fish or poultry.

5

THE ROLES OF ACID AND ALKALI IN THE BODY

ALKALINE RESERVE

In virtually every section of this book, we refer to the body's "alkaline reserve." This concept is vital to understanding the underlying relationship between nutrition and health.

Neutralizing minerals stored throughout the body make up the alkaline reserve. One of the most important of these minerals is sodium. Most of the reserves are stored in the liver to be called upon for use as necessary. As with any reserve, when portions are used or consumed, the supply must either be replenished or the reserve will be diminished and ultimately depleted.

The resources of the alkaline reserve can be thought of as the funds in a checking account. If there is $500 in the account and you write checks on that account, the balance will drop. One check of $500 or five hundred checks of $1 each will deplete the account completely if additional funds are not deposited.

The alkaline reserve of the human physical system works in essentially the same way. If more sodium is required to neutralize acid in the body than is returned to the system through diet, the body will be forced to tap into its alkaline reserve. The body always does what it needs to do to maintain homeostasis — the body never makes a mistake!

There are, basically, two types of substances that make up the alkaline reserve: 1) bicarbonate ions, and 2) fixed alkaline reserves of sodium, potassium, and calcium as primary alkaline minerals, with iron and magnesium as secondary sources. Bicarbonate ions are unable to function in the bicarbonate buffer system unless sodium, potassium, or calcium is present. These minerals have the ability to neutralize acid build-up and are available only through vegetables and fruits.

The body is able to claim alkaline minerals from fruits and vegetables and use them immediately to neutralize acid or store them as part of the alkaline reserve. The liver is probably the greatest single storehouse of minerals although every cell of the body shares this ability. Sodium is stored predominantly in the liver and muscle tissue, while calcium is found in the greatest concentration in the bones.

When cooked protein is consumed, acid ash remains. Although animal protein and milk contain some alkaline minerals, there are not nearly enough to neutralize the strong inorganic acids that result from protein digestion. If these alkaline elements are not replenished by a constant supply of fruits and vegetables in the diet, the body is forced to use alkaline minerals from its reserve in the liver, muscles, and bones.

It is essential to life that some form of buffering takes place since cells produce acid during glycolysis — the process of breaking down glucose into smaller compounds that yield energy the body can use. Alkaline minerals are integral parts of the bicarbonate and phosphate buffer systems that neutralize this and other acids. If the buffering minerals are continuously "spent" without being replaced, as with the checking account, the reserve will be depleted, the body will become increasingly acid and the way will be paved for the onset of a chronic degenerative disease.

The status of the alkaline reserve can be determined by monitoring the pH of urine and saliva. A urine pH reading of 7.0 or above would appear to indicate adequate reserves, but for a patient who is on a consistently high protein diet, this reading usually indicates that the alkaline reserve has been depleted. Consideration of pH in conjunction with other clinical findings is essential.

ACIDITY AND ALKALINITY

In the chapter on pH, we describe the potential of hydrogen as an indicator of the level of acidity or alkalinity of a substance and discuss how this affects the various systems in the body and physiological equilibrium. The acid-alkaline balance, as referenced by pH levels, plays a major role in maintaining the homeostasis that the body seeks. When most of the cells, glands, organs and systems of the body become predominantly acid, or toxic, the total person suffers the consequences.

Although every cell is naturally alkaline, acid is produced as a by-product of cell function. Prompt elimination of this acid is vital to both the functioning and longevity of the cell. When acid elimination slows, for any reason, acid accumulates causing congestion within the cell. As acid production continues to outstrip acid elimination, a cycle of premature degeneration of the cells is established and perpetuated.

Enzymes are destroyed in a strong acid medium. Enzymes are the regulators of homeostasis and all cells function internally by enzymatic action. These enzymes are very specific and function maximally in a very narrow pH range. The more acid the medium, the less effectively the enzyme will function, which, in turn affects the efficiency of cell performance. Acid is implicated in any disease process in the body; multiple sclerosis, diabetes, arthritis, AIDS, or other manifestations of debilitating disease all flourish in an acid environment.

The faster a cell metabolizes, the more acid it produces. Acid is hydrogen ion concentration — it can be generated by exercise or by the processing of food. Regardless of its origin, acid can have a deleterious affect on the body. In this section we will review the relationship between acidity and alkalinity.

POTENCY OF ACIDS

As we have seen, pH values below 7.0 indicate an acid reaction. A weak acid may be pH 5 or 6; a strong acid pH 1 or 2. However, pH is not the only determinant of the strength of an acid. For example, acetic acid with a pH of 3 is relatively harmless while nitric acid, also with a pH of 3, is corrosive, highly detrimental to the body and can burn tissue. Nitric, sulfuric and other strong acids resulting from the digestion of meat must be neutralized immediately by one of the buffering systems. The difference in potency between acetic and nitric acids lies in the rate of ionization or disassociation of the ions of the compound. Acetic acid is ionized only about 3% while nitric acid is fully ionized; that is, all of the hydrogen ions are immediately available, therefore, they must be dealt with immediately.

It is very important to understand the kinds of acids that the body encounters and how the body handles and eliminates them. For our purposes, two particular types of acid will be discussed: *organic acids* with components that are held together loosely by covalent bonds, and *inorganic acids*, the components of which are held together tightly by strong ionic bonds.

ORGANIC ACIDS

Loosely combined organic acids are easily metabolized by the body. For example, the carbon dioxide resulting from cellular metabolism passes easily through the cell wall where it mixes with water to form a weak carbonic acid. This is carried to the lungs where it is acted upon by the enzyme carbonic anhydrase; carbon dioxide is released and expelled by the lungs in exhalation.

The end products of all organic acids from fruits and vegetables are expelled through the lungs. Organic acids, such as citric acid in oranges and malic acid in apples, contain carbon, hydrogen, and oxygen that can be broken down. Organic acids are metabolized through Krebs Cycle, made into CO_2 which is exhaled, and water which is excreted as urine.

Minerals such as sodium, calcium, potassium, magnesium and iron from fruits and vegetables are available to the body. These minerals in the acids of fruits and vegetables are held together loosely by covalent bonds and have an alkalizing effect. After the organic or volatile acids are metabolized, they are available for use or added to the alkaline reserve. The entire process of metabolizing organic acids causes little stress to the body; in fact, this metabolism helps produce energy the body needs to maintain homeostasis.

It is important to understand that organic acids can be metabolized into elements that can be expelled by the lungs. Carbon dioxide that is exhaled is the result of the metabolism of glucose inside the cell — not of the oxygen inhaled. Inhaled oxygen combines with hydrogen produced from food and is eliminated through the kidneys as water. All of the oxygen that has been inhaled and used by the body eventually leaves the body as water. The carbon dioxide that is exhaled by the lungs is made up of the carbon and oxygen that results from the metabolic process of glycolysis.

INORGANIC ACIDS

Inorganic acids pose a real threat to the body. They are ionically bonded — the elements of the compounds are not easily separated. These acids are also highly ionized — up to 95% of the hydrogen ions are active at one time making these substances highly active, therefore, highly corrosive. Since these acids are ionically bonded, they cannot be metabolized inside the cell, and since they are toxic, the body must neutralize them immediately. This neutralization process requires sodium in order to form an acid salt that can be eliminated by the kidneys. The body can use ammonium as a substitute for sodium on a short-term basis when the sodium is depleted, but when the ammonium cannot supply adequate relief, the body turns to the next best source of neutralizing mineral, calcium from the bones.

A rather involved sequence of events takes place in the body in an effort to neutralize inorganic acid. As the blood becomes acid, the buffer systems are stimulated to act but, as we have seen, the bicarbonate buffer system leads off in the buffering process and sodium must be available for this system to work. Sodium can combine with the hydrogen ions to eliminate them in the form of acid salts from the body.

The digestion of cooked meat yields strong inorganic acids — sulfuric, phosphoric, and nitric. These are highly toxic and must be buffered immediately. The body does this by taking a strong acid and making from it a weak acid and an acid salt. Sodium bicarbonate ($NaHCO_3$) combines with the sulfuric acid (H_2SO_4) produced by the digestion of cooked meat and yields sodium hydrogen sulfate ($NaHSO_4$) as the sodium replaces the hydrogen in H_2SO_4. The reaction can be illustrated as follows: $H_2SO_4 + NaHCO_3 \rightarrow H_2CO_3 + NaHSO_4$. The weak carbonic acid (H_2CO_3) is eliminated by way of the lungs and the acid salt is eliminated by the kidneys.

Carbonic acid is ionized 1-3%. Most of it is transferred to the lungs by the red blood cells. While in the RBC, carbonic acid (H_2CO_3) is converted into carbon dioxide (CO_2) and water (H_2O) with the aid of the enzyme carbonic anhydrase. Carbon dioxide and water can then be eliminated by the lungs. Carbonic anhydrase also aids in converting carbon dioxide and water into carbonic acid.

As we shall see in our discussion of excess protein in Chapter Seven, when the blood is too acid and needs bicarbonate for buffering, bicarbonate (HCO_3-). However, when sodium is not available to be combined with the bicarbonate, ammonium (NH_4) made from excess ammonia can substitute for the sodium in the bicarbonate buffer system, forming the acid salt ammonium hydrogen sulfate (NH_4HSO_4).

Recall that the lungs cannot expel the components of inorganic acids. Inorganic acids contain nitrogen, sulfur, or phosphorus that cannot be exhaled. Inorganic acid components are always eliminated through the kidneys.

ACIDOSIS

We are alkaline entities by design but acid generating beings by function. Acid is produced by the parietal cells of the stomach to aid in digestion, and acid is consumed in organic form in fruit. However, other than the stomach, no part of the body should be acid.

Despite this, one of the most widespread and insidious illnesses that plagues our society is acidosis — an accumulation of more acid than the body can effectively process. Patients often initially consult a doctor seeking relief from symptoms of a chronic condition — arthritis, diabetes, emphysema, arteriosclerosis, or cancer. Regardless of the particular symptomatology, all of these conditions originate with an increase in the amount of acid in the body. Acidosis is generally seen by medical science as a part of the pathology of several different diseases including impaired liver function. It is seen often enough to be assumed to be normal, however, acidosis is definitely not normal. It is the forerunner of most, if not all, chronic degenerative diseases including cancer, diabetes, arthritis, and heart disease. These diseases are rampant enough to be considered epidemic in our country.

Acidosis is often a covert condition in that the patient feels good in the early stages of acid accumulation. In fact, he may boast of an exaggerated feeling of well-being and an unusually high level of energy. Unfortunately, this is an inaccurate perception resulting from the "stimulatory" reaction of the body's regulatory systems that are operating in high gear to process the excess acid. Both the good feeling and high energy level will disappear as more acid accumulates. In a continued effort to maintain alkalinity, the neutralizing alkaline reserves are depleted and the liver becomes increasingly congested and is unable to perform its function of detoxification. When the extracellular and intracellular fluids lose their alkalinity, the person is considered to be in a condition of acidosis.

ATTITUDE AND ACIDOSIS

Prolonged periods of acidosis affect not only the physical condition but also the mental and emotional states of patients.

Similarly, mental attitude can affect the physical state. Those who are careful to adhere to the type of diet recommended in this book may limit some of the beneficial effects of the food they eat if they habitually wallow in negative thoughts and attitudes. It is possible for a person to maintain a diet high in fruits and vegetables and still be acid. Regardless of the diet followed, the person who is negative in his outlook on life is acid. Negative thoughts act to stimulate the action of the adrenal glands which in turn speed up the body's metabolic activity. As this occurs, more acid is produced and since the process is continuous, the amount of acid overpowers the alkaline from the good food and the net result is acid. And the cycle can be perpetuated; the more acid we become, the more negative, defensive, argumentative and unpleasant we become. The pessimist who can find nothing good about anything is almost certainly in some degree of acidosis.

SYMPTOMS OF ACIDOSIS

Symptoms of prolonged acidosis that are caused by the consumption of excess protein can easily be mistaken for individual character or personality traits. However, definite attitudes and mannerisms develop as a result of the supercharged internal activity of the body as it works toward ridding itself of the damaging excess acid. The person who is on a high-protein diet moves through a progression of symptoms. Initially, he . . .

- has an exaggerated sense of well-being;
- believes himself to be perfectly well;
- is a high achiever, a "mover and shaker";
- is overly ambitious and restless due to the irritation of the nerves.

Later he . . .

- becomes irritable, ill-tempered, and difficult to please;
- constantly finds fault with everyone and everything;
- sees only the pessimistic side of issues and life;
- can't sleep restfully;
- wakes up as tired in the morning as he was when he went to bed;
- is tired and experiences generalized aches and pains;
- shows signs of "aging" as the body removes alkalizing substances from the muscles then calcium from the bones.

Although everyone who is suffering from acidosis does not experience all of these symptoms, it is helpful for the doctor to be able to correlate some "personality traits" with clinical findings and to recognize indications that the patient's body is overtaxed and headed toward chronic degenerative disease.

RESEARCH AND ACIDOSIS

Researchers have arrived at some interesting though incomplete conclusions from their investigations into the effects acidosis and alkalinity have on the body. In his book, *Arthritis and Folk Medicine*[1], D.C. Jarvis, M.D., outlined a number of things that are beneficial to health; however, he championed some causes for the wrong reasons. For example, as a result of his investigations, he concluded that acid is beneficial. In looking at the alkaline properties involved in cow udder mastitis infections, he concluded that acid combats the alkalinity manifest in this disease.

Mastitis is a condition that impedes milk production and transforms a $2000 milk-producing cow into a $200 non-producing animal in a week. Dr. Jarvis' research involved treating bovine mastitis by introducing large quantities of acid into the body in the form of vinegar which resulted in an improvement of the condition. Dr. Jarvis attributed the improvement to the higher level of acid. He then tried the same experiment substituting phosphoric acid for vinegar but the animal not only showed no improvement, it's condition worsened. He concluded that the acid should be organic to be effective since any organic acid is metabolized into carbon dioxide and water. The significance of the vinegar is that it leaves an alkaline ash of sodium, calcium, potassium, and iron that the animal could use to neutralize the effects of excess acid from the excess dietary protein. The inorganic phosphoric acid, on the other hand, did not leave an alkaline ash, consequently, it did not have the same beneficial results. The results obtained by the vinegar treatment were due to the alkaline ash rather than to an acidifying action. The research was valid but the conclusions were incomplete.

ALKALOSIS

Alkalosis, of course, is the opposite of acidosis, yet some doctors may be perplexed by the similarity of the symptoms of the two conditions. In some instances, the symptoms are identical, particularly those relating to hyperirritability or a volatile personality.

Members of the medical fraternity are accustomed to finding bladder infections associated with alkaline urine, consequently, it is logical for them to assume that alkaline urine is undesirable. However, the alkaline urine they encounter is generally caused by bicarbonate and ammonia which will indeed lead to bladder infection. Seldom will they see urine that is alkaline due to organic minerals in association with a bladder infection.

My observations lead to the conclusion that alkalosis is nothing more than an advanced stage of acidosis. As acid builds up, as the result of excess protein consumption, the body becomes more acid. When this trend continues to the point that the alkaline reserve is gone, the concentration of ammonia increases in the extracellular fluid and bicarbonate ions combine to produce an alkaline urine. It is alkaline because the urine contains ammonia and bicarbonate rather than the neutralizing acid salts that are formed in combination with alkaline reserve minerals. The patient is, indeed, in a state of alkalosis, however, only as a severely advanced degree of acidosis.

Patients whose urine registers an alkaline reaction as a result of a diet high in alkaline-ash producing foods are less likely to suffer from chronic ailments that require frequent trips to the doctor or hospital. Considering the patients usually seen by medical doctors, it is understandable that these physicians would consider acid urine, or acidosis, to be entirely separate and distinct from alkaline urine and alkalosis. My clinical experience, however, indicates that alkalosis in persons who adhere to a high protein diet is acidosis that has progressed to a degree that is a precursor to a pathological condition. The 8.0 pH urine seen in a high-protein consuming patient was 5.5 pH a few years ago; it has advanced from acid to alkaline — not from normal to alkaline. Once again, this interpretation of the implications of acid and alkaline urine is not the generally accepted stance and I welcome results of research by others on this critical facet of the evaluation of patients' health.

6

URINALYSIS INDICATORS

BILIRUBIN

Recognizing that urine contains substances the body is trying to eliminate is the basis for truly appreciating the importance of urinalysis.

Perhaps no other single factor in urinalysis is as clearly linked to nutrition as is bilirubin in the urine. Its presence indicates a problem that can be corrected only by revising nutrition habits. When bilirubin is in the urine in any amount, it is pathological; it indicates that the liver is unable to function correctly and that the kidneys are acting as a detoxification backup system. The liver, the largest internal organ of the body, can lose up to 70% of its functioning capacity before symptoms become apparent; consequently, finding bilirubin in the urine can be significant.

The liver performs many functions related to detoxification. Any normal substance can become toxic to the body if it is located outside of its area of function or if it is concentrated excessively. Most harmful substances are detoxified by the liver and eliminated in the stool; but when the detoxification system of the liver becomes overloaded, for any reason, the kidneys attempt to eliminate abnormal or excessive concentrations of substances.

Bilirubin, a product of the breakdown of red blood cells (RBC), is normal to the blood — it is abnormal to the urine. This section explains the origin, function, and method of elimination of bilirubin.

When an RBC has become fragile, after about 120 days, it is phagocytized by the reticuloendothelial cells. The heme (non-protein portion) is split from the globin (protein) molecule and the porphyrin ring is open at one of the methane bridges. This yields a chain of pyrrole nuclei which is the basic structure of bile pigment.[1] The iron and globin released by the breakdown of the RBCs is transported back to the respective pools of the liver and spleen for storage and reuse.

The first pigment formed, biliverdin, is quickly reduced to bilirubin. As the bilirubin molecule circulates in the blood, it becomes attached to an albumin molecule which renders it insoluble in water as it is transported to the liver. High elevations of this "free bilirubin" are seen in a hemolytic type jaundice which is characterized by excessive RBC destruction.

When the free bilirubin reaches the liver, the liver cells remove the albumin, and the bilirubin is conjugated primarily with glucuronic acid, again becoming highly water soluble. The volume of this conjugated bilirubin will be elevated in any obstructive form of jaundice. The water soluble bilirubin normally is passed through the canaliculi of the liver and secreted into the bile. That portion which is not recycled and reabsorbed passes into the intestine and is further reduced to form urobilinogen.

In order to explain why bilirubin is found in the urine, a review of liver function, jaundice, and the formation and disposition of bile is needed.

THE INTERRELATIONSHIP OF THE LIVER, GALL BLADDER, AND BILE

Bile is made up of alkaline bile salts, bilirubin, cholesterol, fatty acids, lecithin, and minerals. Approximately one liter (1.75 pints) of bile is produced by the liver daily.[2] In a very dilute form as it leaves the liver, the bile is stored and concentrated in the gall bladder.

It is in the gall bladder that water and minerals, including sodium, are reabsorbed. Consequently, when the gall bladder is removed, an important area for reabsorption of sodium is lost. Despite this, the distressed patient who has his gall bladder removed experiences dramatic improvement in digestion and he is again able to eat virtually anything he chooses without suffering adverse symptoms.

Although this observation appears to discredit the non-surgical, holistic philosophy of chiropractic, careful examination of what actually happens will reinforce this philosophy. As chiropractors, we must keep in mind that the body functions to the best of its ability under the conditions imposed upon it.

If we understand that bile is concentrated in the gall bladder, and that cholesterol and bile salts are two of the main constituents of bile, the solution to this mystery begins to unfold as two essential points are considered.

First, bile salts are primarily sodium salts which are water soluble and remain in solution. Second, if the bile salt-to-cholesterol ratio of the bile is maintained, the concentrated gall bladder bile will remain liquid and pass into the duodenum on demand. However, if this ratio becomes unbalanced, the bile begins to precipitate and gall stones begin to form. Gall bladder contractions on hard stones that cause mild to severe obstruction can be extremely painful. Obviously, removing the gall bladder eliminates this source of pain for the patient, but the question remains: "How and why should the removal of an organ cause digestion to improve?" The answer to this question lies in the delicate intra- and extracellular balances that must be maintained.

First, an observation: Removal of the gall bladder of a healthy individual does not improve his digestion; only a patient with gall bladder distress will experience relief of symptoms.

As noted previously, bile is produced by the liver then stored and concentrated in the gall bladder. When we remove a distressed gall bladder, we remove the ability to reabsorb sodium and bicarbonate into the blood. In a functioning gall bladder, sodium is reabsorbed from the liver bile changing it from a natural alkaline bile of pH 8.5 to an unnatural acid bile of pH 4.5. If the gall bladder is removed, the sodium remains in the liver bile allowing the bile to maintain its alkaline nature, and this alkaline bile then passes directly into the duodenum allowing normal digestion to occur. The duodenum is supposed to be alkaline in the digestive process.

BILE SALTS

In the normal function of the digestive system, alkaline bile salts serve two primary purposes: 1) they aid in the emulsification of fats, fatty acids, cholesterol and other lipids, and 2) they help in the absorption of digested fats into the circulation. Bile salts themselves are reabsorbed and recycled. Reabsorption takes place in the jejunum, perhaps as frequently as twice each meal. This process may not be normal, but for patients on high fat diets, it has become necessary. Some of the bile salts make their way into the large intestine where further reabsorption occurs if the pH of this environment is alkaline. If the large intestine is acid, reabsorption is impaired and acid crystals are formed.[3]

Without bile salts, fatty acids are lost into the stool which leads not only to a deficiency of essential fatty acids but also to a deficiency of the fat soluble vitamins A, D, E, and K.[4]

HOW GALL STONES BECOME NECESSARY

We have noted that organic material is covalently bonded. Bile is over 98% organic in nature, and the body uses only covalent substances in natural physiology. The nuclear magnetic resonance of inorganic sodium is different from that of living, covalent sodium found in living systems, and we have seen that the body does not effectively or efficiently use the inorganic sodium found in table salt (NaCl). However, as discussed in the pH section, the blood must remain alkaline. If the body's alkaline reserve is deficient, bicarbonate and sodium are reabsorbed into the blood from the gall bladder in an attempt to maintain the reserves. Sodium is then available as organic-covalent sodium salt compounds in bile salts to be reabsorbed into the blood and used again in the buffering processes. This upsets the bile salt-to-cholesterol ratio which reduces the liquidity of the concentrated gall bladder bile and interferes with the removal of cholesterol from the gall bladder. Most gall stones have a core of cholesterol, bilirubin, and protein.[5]

It becomes obvious that the body, in its infinite wisdom, will reabsorb sodium from the gall bladder in an attempt to maintain life-sustaining alkaline blood even though the bile salt-to cholesterol ratio is upset and gall stones may be formed. The body's priority is to preserve life — it is more important to maintain the blood pH at 7.4 than to leave the sodium in the gall bladder to prevent the formation of stones in the gall bladder.

It is now apparent that gall stones are the product of a process that has become necessary for survival, yet the removal of the gall bladder results in an apparent improvement of digestion.

When the gall bladder has been removed, the body has lost an important source from which sodium can be reclaimed, and the muscles become the next source of supply. When this source (along with the reserves stored in the liver) has been exhausted, the body will utilize calcium as a buffering agent in an attempt to maintain adequate alkaline reserves for natural, normal physiology.

Even though digestion is improved temporarily, the long-term effect of removing the gall bladder is that health in general must continue downhill unless the diet is changed. An acid-ash producing diet was the cause of the problem in the first place — we must treat the cause to reach lasting overall improvement in health.

JAUNDICE

While bile serves in many vital physiological functions, its appearance outside of normal functional areas can be an indicator of serious problems. If it collects in the skin, jaundice (or icterus) results.

Jaundice may be evident in intra- and extracellular hepatic obstruction, serum and infectious hepatitis, infectious mononucleosis, drug or alcohol induced hepatitis, cirrhosis, tumors, and septicemia.

The two primary types of jaundice are hemolytic and obstructive.

Hemolytic Jaundice

In hemolytic jaundice, the red blood cells are destroyed at a rate faster than the liver can process them, however, bilirubin will not be present in the urine. The liver is unable to adequately conjugate the bilirubin because of excess RBC destruction, therefore, the bilirubin is not water soluble and cannot be excreted by the kidneys. In this situation, a patient will have yellow skin and yellow eyes but will not have bilirubin in the urine. In hemolytic jaundice, the stool will probably be a normal dark color and of normal odor.

Obstructive Jaundice

In obstructive jaundice, bile is produced normally but its normal excretory pathway (beginning in the liver and ending in the duodenum) is obstructed or blocked. Although this obstruction can occur anywhere along the pathway, the most common location is the gall bladder.

Obstruction due to liver cell congestion is becoming more common and deserves special attention. Liver congestion can occur when the blood becomes so toxic that the liver cannot detoxify (or clean) it rapidly enough. When this occurs, the liver cells retain fluid (mainly water) in an attempt to dilute the toxins until they can be metabolized and the waste material eliminated in the bile.

This dilution back-up system works well while adequate alkalinity is maintained. When adequate alkalinity is not available, further dilution occurs until the cells become engorged with fluid, rupture the canaliculi of the cell, and bile spills directly into the blood stream. Since this bile has been conjugated in the liver before spilling into the blood, it is now water soluble and can be excreted by the kidneys and discharged in the urine. If the amount is too great for the kidneys to excrete, the excess is deposited in the skin turning it yellow.

The toxicity or congestion that caused the liver cells to swell can originate with diet or with toxic fat released during a fast; the most common factor is diet — more protein has been consumed than the body needs. If congestion is due to excess protein, the diet must be changed drastically; if the congestion occurs during a cleansing fast, the speed of cleansing must be reduced. Ordinarily, reintroducing carbohydrates into the diet through fruit or cooked vegetables brings the patient out of ketosis caused by a water or juice fast and is sufficient to slow the release of toxic fat and to eliminate bilirubin from the urine.

Any amount of bilirubin in the urine is pathological and immediate steps to eliminate it should be taken. Bilirubin in trace, or to a measurement of +1, is not critical but must be monitored a minimum of every other day. A +2 or +3 bilirubin level must be checked daily until it declines. Bilirubin in the urine that is caused by drugs or a toxic diet is treated most effectively by a diet of raw fresh juice, preferably carrot juice.

If the bilirubin appears in the urine due to limited carbohydrate intake, such as occurs during a fast, carbohydrate intake must be increased in the form of cooked vegetables until the bilirubin level is reduced.

Regardless of the cause, a patient with obstructive jaundice will have bilirubin in the urine and may have yellow skin, yellow eyes, and a light colored, foul-smelling stool. Patients with hemolytic jaundice will also have yellow skin and eyes, but may not have bilirubin in the urine.

As chiropractors, we need to be aware of and able to identify a very important third type of jaundice — dietary.

Dietary Jaundice

A third type of jaundice that may cause patients some alarm is dietary jaundice. If an excessive amount of carrot juice is consumed, the skin will turn yellow but the sclera of the eyes will remain white and there will be no sign of bilirubin in the urine. Yellow skin and white eyes is not as serious as yellow skin and yellow eyes.

Two to four pints of carrot juice daily will turn the skin of most patients yellow in three weeks. The yellow color is due to excess carotene from the carrot juice being deposited in the skin until the carotene can be properly metabolized. The palms of the hands usually turn yellow first. If the amount of carrot juice is reduced when this initial indication appears, the skin usually will not continue to yellow.

Dietary jaundice is not a pathological condition. The key indicator of the pathological nature of jaundice is the whites of the eyes. As long as they remain white, regardless of the color of the skin, the patient is in control. If a person is drinking enough carrot juice to turn the skin yellow, there is a good possibility that rapid cleansing of the body is taking place. If this cleansing is too rapid for the liver to accommodate the detoxification requirements, congestive jaundice could occur and bilirubin will appear in the urine. If this happens, the patient should reduce the carrot juice intake significantly and eat cooked vegetables for three to seven days, or until the bilirubin disappears from the urine. Hans A. Nieper, M.D., has stated that if a seriously ill patient cannot experience a yellowing of the skin, his chances of survival are greatly diminished.[6]

The following chart summarizes symptoms that can be attributed to the three different types of jaundice.

BILIRUBIN—JAUNDICE SUMMARY CHART

Type of Jaundice	Free Bilirubin in Blood	Conjugated Bilirubin in Blood	Skin	Eyes	Stool Odor	Stool Color
OBSTRUCTIVE Usually Gall Bladder or Duct	Low	High	Yellow	Yellow	Foul	Light
HEMOLYTIC	High	Low	Yellow	Yellow	Normal	Normal
DIETARY Not Pathological	Normal	Normal	Yellow	White	Normal	Normal

In all types of jaundice, a blood profile is helpful. Liver cells have specific enzymes that perform specific functions. When extensive liver cell destruction occurs, for whatever reason, excessive amounts of enzymes will be present in the blood. Since this is not a manual on blood, we will only mention enzymes such as SGPT and SGOT as specific liver enzymes that could be in elevated levels in liver problems of all kinds.

KETONES

When determining the optimum rate of dietary change a patient can tolerate, pH and ketones should be considered. A trace of ketones in the urine along with a trace of bilirubin could indicate that the liver is cleansing the patient at maximum tolerance. This situation must be monitored very carefully to assure that the level of ketones does not rise above a trace — the point at which maximum cleansing and healing can take place safely.

As liver function improves and the alkaline reserve begins to accumulate there should be no bilirubin present and a moderate level of ketones can be tolerated. If the urine pH can be kept at 6.0 or above, there is very little danger that this patient will go into ketotic or diabetic coma. However, if ketones are present in the urine along with glucose and an acid level of pH 5.5 or below, there is danger of the onset of diabetic acidosis that, if untreated, could lead to diabetic coma.

A disease that chiropractors are seeing with increasing frequency is candidiasis, a yeast condition that thrives in an acid medium. Medical chemical therapy has not been very effective in treating this condition.

The most effective treatment for a patient with candidiasis is to reduce the carbohydrate intake to the point at which a trace of ketones appears in the urine. This can usually be done by having the patient consume only two to four bananas per day, or an equivalent amount of a comparable fruit. The patient should be closely monitored since the amount of fruit required to achieve this trace of ketones will vary depending upon the patient's exercise level. A good indication of a healthy healing environment is one in which the urine shows a trace of ketones and a pH of 6.0 or above.

UROBILINOGEN

It was stated earlier that some of the bilirubin finds its way to the large intestine. Here it is hydrolyzed by intestinal bacteria into urobilin (the pigment that passes into the stool giving it the characteristic color) and urobilinogen.

Urobilinogen is a colorless substance that is reabsorbed into the circulation from the large intestine. It is returned to the liver through the portal vein. When urobilinogen is found in the urine, it means that there is a high level in the blood which further indicates that high levels of bilirubin are being formed. Logic would indicate that the body has a constructive use for reabsorbed urobilinogen, but as yet, this purpose has not become evident. In essence, we can say that the liver was already in trouble before urobilinogen was found in the urine.

Monitoring the level of urobilinogen, in conjunction with consideration of the amount of bilirubin, provides indicators as to how fast the patient can change to a more healthful diet.

According to laboratory manuals, a small amount of urobilinogen is normal. We must consider this in the light of the concepts of Normal, Natural, and Necessary. It certainly isn't normal, but undoubtedly it is necessary for specific patients at specific times. We must always remember that everything the body does is intelligent, correct, and appropriate.

INDICAN

My experience has shown that toxicity is the first step toward any of the chronic degenerative diseases. Indican found in the urine in any amount indicates toxicity in the body.

When indican is present in the urine, the protein level will be elevated and the urine will have a green or blue-green tint. Indican is a compound formed by the decomposition of the essential amino acid tryptophan that is normally digested in the small intestine. When the incompletely digested tryptophan arrives in the large intestine, indole is formed and absorbed by the blood and then further modified to indican by the liver. If there is a deficiency of pancreatic enzymes, digestion is incomplete. Pancreatic enzymes will supplement the deficient pancreatic secretions. Betaine hydrochloride will also be needed since a highly toxic body is unable to produce adequate HCl or pancreatic enzymes. These supplements should be reduced as the toxicity level decreases.

A +4 indican level in the urine does not dictate the onset of cancer, but it does indicate that the patient is a candidate for chronic degenerative disease. With a +3 level, arthritic symptoms can be suspected, and the indican level may also be elevated in obstructive jaundice.

When a patient is monitored and the indican level in his urine goes from a +4 to neutral, this is clinical evidence that this patient has improved his diet and now has a good possibility of recovering — it may take a month or two, but it can be the first step to reversing many chronic degenerative diseases.

Although indican may be found in conjunction with bilirubin and urobilinogen, there is no significant correlation. The level of indican in the urine indicates the level of toxicity; the levels of bilirubin, urobilinogen, and pH are guides as to just how fast dietary changes can be made.

Remember that toxicity in the blood can come from a current junk food diet, from too much protein, or from a cleansing fast that releases the toxins stored in fat.

7

PROTEIN — EXCESSIVE VS. ESSENTIAL

PROTEIN

This section looks at how protein interacts in the digestive system; how it can alter the pH level of the body; the effect it has on the body's reserves of the neutralizing elements sodium and calcium; and ways we can help patients combat the system-damaging effects that accrue from consuming more protein than their bodies can effectively process.

Protein is credited with being essential to achieving and maintaining good health, a high energy level, and weight control. Even the name, taken from the Greek word "protos" meaning "first," demonstrates the long-held theory that protein is the chief constituent of living matter.

Proteins are highly complex nitrogenous compounds found in all living matter — from the most simple albumin to the intricate genetic codes of DNA, proteins provide amino acids that are necessary for growth and repair of animal tissue. Enzymes and most hormones are primarily protein. Protein is essential for building new cells, transmitting genetic material from one cell to another, and is vital to the proper functioning and regulation of the many systems that make up the human body.

PROTEIN REQUIREMENTS

Our bodies need protein to build new tissue and repair injured tissue; **the importance of protein in our diets cannot be overemphasized**. However, the quantities generally recommended as the amount needed to keep us energetic, well-nourished, and healthy are considerably higher than the amount actually needed or healthful.

The public has been conditioned to believe that large quantities of protein-rich foods, especially beef and dairy products, contribute to our stamina, build strong muscles, and generally promote good health. However, when we consider that the composition of mother's milk is approximately 1.5% protein we can see that vast quantities of protein are not essential to growth and the development of new cells. In addition, other authorities have revised their recommendations and advise that protein should make up only about 2.5% of our dietary intake.[1]

Two and one-half percent is far less protein than the quantities recommended by leading nutritionists. However, this percentage is much more in keeping with the level found in human milk that is consumed following birth when cell production is most rapid. Infants double their birth weight in the first six months on a diet that consists almost entirely of milk that is not only 1.0 to 1.5% protein but also alkaline in reaction.

Protein requirement recommendations are based on studies using white rats that produce milk of approximately 9% protein. This high percentage of protein is consistent with the rapid growth rate and comparatively short maturation period of rats. However, the protein requirements are far different for a species that takes approximately eighteen years to reach maturity.

To illustrate how attitudes concerning protein requirements have changed over the years, in the latter part of the nineteenth century, 118 grams (about 4 oz.) of protein per day was the amount nutritionists recommended for healthful diet. By 1974, this amount had been adjusted down to 56 grams (about 2 oz.) per day. Today, some authorities believe than an adult human can live well on as little as 20 grams (2/3 oz.) of protein per day.[2] Even more startling, evidence from clinical research indicates that vegetable protein is more beneficial and more effectively assimilated than is animal protein![3] Yet ours is a steak and potatoes culture — or at least a hamburger and french fries culture. Many Americans feel that a meal is not complete without meat of some sort.

My research has shown that excess animal protein consumption adversely impacts our bodies in ways that are subtle but quantitatively definable. Clinical evaluations reveal that patients who eat large quantities of meat generate high levels of acid that must be neutralized before being eliminated from the body. As we shall see, on a high-protein diet, very acid urine will be produced initially, and if high protein intake continues, a very alkaline urine will eventually result. However, these acidic-alkaline responses are not capricious functions of the body; rather, they are attempts by the body both to maintain the slightly alkaline pH that is most conducive to homeostatic function and to rid itself of the end product of excessive protein consumption — acid ash.

THE PROTEIN CONNECTION

In an earlier chapter, we discussed how ash is formed, and we listed foods that produce acid ash and alkaline ash. To recap, ash is a product of digestion of both meat and vegetables. Animal protein, dairy products, eggs, and grains leave an acid ash, while fruits and vegetables, for the most part, leave an alkaline ash. Some foods such as white sugar and other processed or synthetic foods leave no ash but have an acidifying effect on the body.

High-protein foods produce strong inorganic acids, such as nitric, sulfuric, and phosphoric, and also leave acid ash — all of which require alkalizing minerals for neutralization. Highly refined carbohydrates, characteristic of convenience foods, result in smaller quantities of inorganic acid ash that require less of the alkaline reserve to neutralize. The end products of carbohydrate metabolism, water and carbon dioxide, can easily be eliminated by the lungs and kidneys without further neutralization. The acid residue of excess animal and grain protein, on the other hand, must be neutralized before being eliminated from the body, and this neutralization requires the body to expend valuable sodium as a buffering agent.

This is not to imply that high carbohydrate foods such as junk food are desirable or that they constitute a nutritious diet; it does illustrate, however, that different types of food produce different situations with which the body must deal. The standard American and junk food diets will both lead to chronic degenerative disease; the difference is the route taken and the rate of acceleration of disease.

We have stated that the body attempts to maintain a metabolic homeostatic balance and a slightly alkaline pH despite the acid ash produced by excess dietary protein. In our discussion of pH, we have referred to Guyton's implication of pH as the single most important factor in maintaining homeostasis. Every part of the body, with the exception of the stomach, should be alkaline. To maintain homeostasis when excess acid has been produced, the body uses built-in bicarbonate, phosphate, or protein buffer systems in an attempt to sustain a normal, slightly alkaline pH. The nitric, sulfuric, or phosphoric acids that are produced as a result of the digestion of meat increase acidity and cause stress as the body attempts to neutralize and eliminate the acids. Normally, the strong inorganic nitric and sulfuric acids produced by protein metabolism are combined with sodium to produce sodium acid salts that would show the urine to be a highly acid 4.0 to 5.5 pH.

Yet a person can eat a big steak at night and the following morning's analysis will indicate a slightly alkaline urine pH of

8. Although this appears to be a contradiction of the premise that too much protein depletes the alkaline reserve, this paradox can be explained.

Unlike other foods, protein causes the parietal cells of the gastric mucosa to secrete hydrochloric acid (HCl). The HCl is made from carbonic acid (H_2CO_3). When one part hydrogen is removed from the carbonic acid, bicarbonate (HCO_3-), an alkaline substance, remains. If the body's sodium supply has been depleted or seriously diminished, the bicarbonate ions (that would ordinarily combine with sodium to be reabsorbed) pass into the urine which then has an alkaline reading. However, had the bicarbonate ions followed the preferred course and been recombined with sodium molecules and reabsorbed by the kidney, the bicarbonate would not be eliminated and the urine would be acidic. Consequently, an alkaline urine pH for a person whose diet ordinarily consists of meat and other high-protein foods, indicates that the alkaline reserve has been depleted, the bicarbonate cannot be reabsorbed by the kidney, and the bicarbonate and ammonia are passing into the urine giving the urine an alkaline reading.

Recall that we identified protein as complex nitrogenous substances. In essence, the problems generated by a high protein diet lie in the compensations the body must make to cast off the excess nitrogen. When there is only a moderate amount of protein to be processed, the body is able to eliminate nitrogen as urea, a neutral salt, which is produced by each cell in normal metabolism. As meat consumption continues and more acid ash must be disposed of, the body eliminates the excess nitrogen as uric acid — a condition associated with gout. As still more meat is consumed, even more acid is produced and the body must resort to buffering the acids by taking sodium from the alkaline reserve to produce acid salts that are eliminated in the urine. When the toxic load becomes too great and the alkaline reserves are depleted, the body will rid itself of excess nitrogen by eliminating it directly into the urine first as ammonia then as protein and ultimately as both protein and ammonia.

CHAIN OF EVENTS CAUSED BY EXCESS PROTEIN

Sodium taken from alkaline reserve
   — produces acid salts to be eliminated.   Acid urine

↓

Nitrogen eliminated naturally as urea.   Acid urine

↓

Nitrogen eliminated as uric acid.   Acid urine

↓

Alkaline reserve depleted.   Acid urine

↓

Nitrogen eliminated directly as
   ammonium acid salt.   Acid urine

↓

Nitrogen eliminated directly as ammonia
   in urine.   Alkaline urine

↓

Bicarbonate eliminated directly as
   ammonia in urine.   Alkaline urine

↓

Calcium starts being used as secondary
   buffer.   Alkaline urine

↓

Protein, ammonia, and bicarbonate
   in urine   Alkaline urine

This chain of events not only illustrates how the alkaline reserve is depleted but also why a high-protein consuming patient can register an alkaline urine pH although his entire system is acidotic.

We state throughout this study that excess acids in the body are neutralized by sodium from the alkaline reserve. When these reserves have been tapped for a long period of time, the sodium level is reduced — the bank balance goes down. When the sodium level is too low, the body will excrete ammonia (NH_3) directly into the urine, giving the urine an alkaline pH. This is an ingenious way for the body to eliminate both excess nitrogen and excess hydrogen, but it is not Natural, it is not Normal — it is absolutely Necessary!

When excess protein is consumed, the body must deal with the acid component of protein, excess hydrogen ions ($H+$), as well as nitrogen (N). Neither of these substances can be eliminated through the lungs; they must be eliminated through the urinary tract. Each time sulfuric or nitric acid must be neutralized, the body loses vital sodium in the formation of an acid salt that can be eliminated in the urine. The body will attempt to conserve or replace this physiological sodium with the ammonium radical (NH_4+) in the formation of an acid salt (NH_4HSO_4).

Recall that elimination of excess nitrogen is necessary if excess protein is consumed. We need nitrogen in our protein, but we don't need too much of it. The nitrogen can be eliminated as an acid nitrate salt or as ammonia, which is alkaline. When the bicarbonate and phosphate buffer systems are overtaxed, we have another backup system that is a by-product of the excess nitrogen that the body is trying to eliminate. Ammonia plus the hydrogen ions from excess acid-ash food consumption yield the ammonium radical that can substitute for a lack of sodium in the bicarbonate buffer system. However, this system is available only on a short-term basis.

The body makes ammonia in the kidneys and most other cells. The body takes a waste product of nitrogen that it must eliminate and uses it to neutralize its own negative acidifying effects. What a marvelous system!

However, this system will also become overloaded and the sodium will ultimately be lost directly as excessive acid salts are formed. If all of the available sodium is expended, the body will utilize calcium as the best alternative to neutralize the acid. Bones provide the most readily available supply of this buffering material, and after a prolonged period of using this source, osteoporosis will result. If 47 grams of protein are consumed per day, the body will lose more calcium than it can assimilate regardless of the diet or supplementation.[4] Protein continues to act as a stimulus to remove calcium from the bones and, as the necessity for processing acid ash persists, virtually every organ and system of the body will exhibit some adverse reaction.

Neutralizing minerals are found throughout the body but the liver is the major storehouse for sodium. If adequate alkaline reserves are not available to meet the demands on the liver, it will use the sodium available from its own cells. When these cells then cease to function, they die, scarred tissue characteristic of cirrhosis is formed, and the liver shuts down a portion of its activity.[5] The liver will not produce inferior bile! There is no obvious problem initially since liver reserves are great enough to allow up to 70% loss of functional capacity without the deficiencies being apparent.

As the liver continues to be affected, the body's defenses against disease are reduced and chronic degenerative diseases, such as arthritis, diabetes, emphysema, cancer, AIDS, and circulatory disorders have a fertile acid-medium field in which to become established. My research and experience indicate that cancer cells can proliferate in an acid medium or in a medium that is alkaline due to the presence of bicarbonate and ammonia. Both of these environments are the result of the same process — the long-term efforts of the body to process excess protein. Regardless of the specific chronic degenerative disease that results, it can be attributed to alkaline reserve depletion brought about by sustained protein consumption intensified by long-term insufficiencies of fruits and vegetables in the diet.

Over a period of years, the kidneys will become incapable of reabsorbing vital organic material, and the urine will be highly alkaline due to loss of kidney function rather than to dietary habits. Ammonia and bicarbonate in the urine contribute to a high incidence of bladder irritations and infections that are often seen in conjunction with wasting diseases. Since most people are not exclusively carnivores, the process of sodium depletion, calcium loss, and the onset of chronic degenerative disease takes a slow, insidious course. We have been referring to excess protein that is consumed along with other foods. Assuming that our patients eat vegetables and fruits in at least moderate amounts, the beneficial properties of these foods will serve to offset the destructive effects of animal protein, but only to a limited degree.

THE EFFECT OF EXCESS PROTEIN ON CELLS

Excess protein consumption over a long period stresses all body functions. It can affect the very essence of our existence — the cells. Relatively recent technology has revealed that cells are able to, and do, store protein. We noted in Chapter Three that when excess protein is stored in cells it interferes with the normal cellular osmotic action. Cells take in and retain more water to dilute the acid build-up caused by the excess protein. Water retention is the least harmful alternative for the body when the acid level is too high. The increased level of water causes more congestion in the cells, the osmotic balance is altered and the pressure gradient is changed; however, these undesirable conditions are preferable to the consequences that would otherwise be associated with higher acid. Unfortunately, fluid retention is often treated with a diuretic which forces the body to lose water, which in effect concentrates the acid, raising it again to a dangerous level. The body does *not* retain more water than it needs in its attempt to maintain homeostasis.

THE RELATIONSHIP BETWEEN PROTEIN AND MINERAL DEFICIENCIES

Most patients would take issue with the premise that they are deficient in sodium and would jump at the chance to justify their use of table salt. Few patients are aware of the difference between the strong ionically bonded mineral table salt (NaCl) that resists being separated into sodium and chloride ions in the body, and the loosely, covalently bonded sodium found in fruits and vegetables. It is important that patients understand that table salt will not replenish a sodium deficiency that is the result of excess animal protein consumption. The body cannot use salt, nor can it use the sodium in salt. The salt dissolves in the water of the body and becomes $Na+$ ions and $Cl-$ ions. Even though these ions are separated, the electrical attraction between them is stronger than the body can effectively overcome.

Similarly, patients should understand that adults can develop a calcium deficiency by drinking cow's milk. Cow's milk differs from human milk in composition. Both kinds contain alkalizing minerals, along with some acidifying components. However, human milk contains a far greater proportion of alkaline to acid — about 3:1, which is close to the physiological calcium to phosphorous ratio. Cow's milk, on the other hand, contains these components in a ratio that is close to 1:1. By drinking cow's milk, the delicate mineral balance is upset. In an effort to bring the alkaline to acid ratio to a more nearly normal level, the body will withdraw calcium from the only available source of alkalizing minerals — the bones. Cow's milk, in effect, initiates a stimulus that results in calcium being withdrawn from the bones; so we can see how consumption of large quantities of milk could lead to osteoporosis.

Sudden reduction in meat and dairy products consumption may cause some patients to experience muscle cramps that can be attributed to a change in the availability of calcium. If the alkaline reserve is depleted and a high protein diet has provided the stimulus for withdrawing calcium from the bones, when the dietary protein is eliminated, the calcium extraction stimulus is also eliminated. Even though the patient may be eating more fruits and vegetables, the patient's enzymatic processes have not had time to personalize the dietary calcium, therefore that source of calcium is unavailable and the body has neither the stimulus to withdraw calcium from the bones nor the ability to utilize the dietary calcium. The patient is now experiencing a true calcium deficiency and muscle cramps can result. The relationship between excess protein, calcium deficiency, and osteoporosis is discussed in greater detail in Chapter Eight.

The patient who has reached the point of experiencing muscle cramps may be given acid-ash producing foods again until the cramps subside. Then he must be alkalized gradually by adding fruits and vegetables to his diet. Saliva pH readings act as a guide as to how fast this can be done.

When treating any of the many symptoms of acidosis, keep in mind that stimuli should not be taken away suddenly — fruits and vegetables should be added to the diet by degrees so that the body can become accustomed to new patterns of food.

VEGETABLES PROVIDE PROTEIN

Contrary to common belief, most vegetables contain the protein, essential amino acids, and iron necessary to replenish cells and maintain healthy cellular function — the basis by which our bodies live. To cite a few examples of protein-rich vegetables, cabbage, broccoli, celery, and asparagus contain approximately 1.5% protein, a cup of green beans about 2.4%, and kidney beans offer approximately the same amount of protein as pork. The human body does not need animal protein to grow, replenish cells or to function. Meat is an acquired taste (as are many other common dietary items such as salt, sugar, coffee, pepper) that can be habit forming.

When vegetables and fruits constitute the major dietary protein source, the ash remaining, after the digestive process has extracted the nutrients, contains alkaline minerals that help the body to maintain the healthful slightly alkaline pH level at which it functions most efficiently and effectively. Since toxic acids are minimal in a predominantly vegetable and fruit diet, high levels of sodium are not needed for neutralization and the sodium level is replenished and maintained. With an adequate supply of sodium to act as the primary buffer, the secondary source of neutralization, calcium, remains in the bones. A final benefit of altering the type of protein we furnish our systems is that the delicate osmotic balance is restored to the cells and normal cellular function resumes.

Confirmed high-protein advocates may express concern that a diet of fruits and vegetables will lead to energy loss since protein has traditionally been equated with furnishing energy. Our research indicates that protein is, in fact, a negative energy source. Each process involved in assimilating and eliminating protein requires an expenditure of energy. More energy is required to digest protein than the protein yields, and the kidneys expend energy in processing excess protein for elimination.

Energy is lost each time excessive protein is introduced into the digestive system. Protein is never a direct energy source — glucose is the fuel that provides energy. Although protein can be converted into glucose by the process of glyconeogenesis, more energy is used in the conversion than the resulting glucose yields. The "energy" that is thought to be generated by eating large amounts of protein is due to stimulation as the body responds to the processing. Protein is one of the most powerful stimulants to the body other than drugs. We do not ordinarily think of protein as a stimulant, but in large quantities it has long-term stimulatory effects. A cup of coffee may act as a stimulant for about an hour, but a steak will stimulate a person for four to five hours. While the body processes the steak the person generally feels good, however, this feeling is the result of energy-consuming stimulation that can be misinterpreted as energy.

We must bear in mind that the compensations the body is forced to make to accommodate to excess protein are necessary. The body does not know how to be sick; it can only react to the stimuli presented and do the best it can with what it has to work with. The responses required of the body to handle excess protein are neither Normal nor Natural, but they are certainly Necessary.

SUMMARY

Excess protein consumption causes stress to the body. It results in the formation of strong acids — sulfuric, nitric, and phosphoric — that must be neutralized and eliminated. This neutralization process requires a plentiful supply of sodium which is a large portion of the alkaline reserve. The alkaline reserve is maintained by a diet consisting predominantly of fruits and vegetables. If excessive amounts of protein are consumed, more sodium is withdrawn from the reserves than is replaced, and eventually the sodium is depleted. The body then turns to the next best alkalizing mineral, calcium, which is taken from the bones, ultimately leading to osteoporosis. All of the buffer systems are affected and as the levels of acid and protein rise, cellular congestion occurs, the entire body begins to slow down and chronic degenerative disease soon follows. On a high protein diet, the patient progresses through the phases of more protein, more acid, less sodium, more congestion, and inevitable disease.

Recall that we have been referring to "excess protein." The body needs protein for the development and repair of cells. Meat is one source of this vital substance. However, vegetables also provide all of the nutrients our bodies require. Our diets should be made up mostly of vegetables and fruit with only small amounts of meat, poultry and fish. Our metabolism can accommodate small amounts of meat without serious adverse effects as long as fruits and vegetables are consumed in substantial quantities to provide the loosely bonded sodium required to neutralize acid ash. Although fruits and most vegetables are highly acid in their natural state, the ash produced is alkaline.

Our patients, need to understand the importance of eating less animal protein so that there is less acid to neutralize, and of eating more fruits and vegetables so that the alkaline reserve can be restored. With these curative measures, sodium will again be deposited within the cells, calcium will not be extracted from the bones to act as a buffering agent, buffer systems will work efficiently, excess protein will be reduced, and the osmotic balance will be normalized to permit life-giving cellular function to proceed as intended.

8

CALCIUM, PROTEIN, AND OSTEOPOROSIS

CALCIUM AS A BUFFERING AGENT

Throughout this book, we have emphasized the importance of sodium as the primary, first-called-upon mineral to buffer the acid produced daily by the Standard American Diet. We have described how sodium is lost through the kidneys as an acid salt of sodium hydrogen phosphate or sodium hydrogen sulfate, and how the sodium of the alkaline reserve is depleted if it is not replenished through foods that provide adequate dietary organic sodium.

As this process continues, sodium reserves are diminished to a level that cannot adequately buffer accumulated acid, and the body uses calcium to assure a life-sustaining buffering process. The body functions only in the present; it does not plan for the future; buffering acid is an immediate need that must be met even if it leads to the development of some chronic degenerative disease in the future.

As mentioned in Chapter Seven, when as little as 47 grams of protein a day is consumed, more calcium is lost from the body than is replenished. To relate this amount to a Standard

American Diet, a breakfast of 3.5 oz. each of bacon, fried eggs, and whole wheat toast yields approximately 55 grams of protein — and the main "meat meal" of the day is yet to come. With this quantity of dietary protein to contend with, the sodium supply will almost assuredly be depleted and the secondary buffering source, calcium, will be called upon.

THE EFFECTS OF EXCESS PROTEIN ON CALCIUM LEVELS

Calcium levels in the blood are normally maintained at approximately 9 to 10 milligrams per deciliter (mg/dl).[1] However, as we shall see, even when dietary or supplementary calcium is provided, the body may be able maintain this blood calcium level but it may be unable to use the calcium to neutralize the acidifying effects of excess protein. In order to maintain a level of 9 to 10 mg/dl when usable dietary calcium is not available, the body will withdraw calcium from the bones thereby opening the way to the development of osteoporosis. By understanding this concept, it becomes evident that findings of normal blood calcium levels do not guarantee freedom from osteoporosis. "When a person has a continuing deficiency of calcium in the diet," writes Guyton, " parathyroid hormone often can stimulate enough calcium absorption from the bones to maintain a normal plasma calcium ion concentration for a year or more; but eventually even the bones will run out of calcium."[2]

According to the 1980 revision of the Recommended Daily Dietary Allowances issued by the Food and Nutrition Board, National Academy of Sciences — National Research Council, 800 mg of calcium per day is recommended for most adults. This amount, or any amount, will not be sufficient to prevent the extraction of calcium from the bones as long as acidifying elements in the diet are present in quantities that overwhelm the body's ability to neutralize excessive acid ash. The demand for calcium placed on the body by dietary practices (particularly excess protein consumption) contributes more to the depletion of calcium from the bones than does a deficiency of calcium intake. Even when adequate amounts of calcium are made available to the body, there is a time delay before the calcium can act as a replenishing substance. The body cannot metabolize the calcium fast enough to compensate for the negative effects of excess protein. And, of course, excess protein in the diet imposes other stringent demands upon the resources of the body.

The effect of high protein consumption was the subject of a report in the *American Journal of Clinical Nutrition*. This report states: "Urine calcium excretion is known to be directly correlated with the level of dietary protein intake. In this experiment we examined the persistence of the hypercalciuria induced by the consumption of high protein diets, and the mechanism of the calciuric response. In a 95-day metabolic study, each of six adult male subjects received formula diets supplying 12 g nitrogen or 36 g nitrogen, and approximately 1400 mg calcium per day. Urine calcium increased rapidly and significantly from an average of 191 mg/day on the 12 g nitrogen diet to 277 mg/day on the 36 g nitrogen diet. There was no significant difference in the apparent absorption of calcium, so that overall calcium balance was -37 mg/day on the 12 g nitrogen diet, and significantly lower at -137 mg/day in subjects consuming the high protein diet. . . . The consumption of high calcium diets is unlikely to prevent the negative calcium balance and probable bone loss induced by the consumption of high protein diets."[3]

CALCIUM LOSS

This same study showed that on a daily diet of 12 grams of nitrogen and 1392 mg of calcium, two-thirds of the subjects were in a negative calcium balance. The report goes on to say: "All of the subjects were in negative calcium balance on the high protein diet, with an average negative balance of 137 mg/day. This rate of calcium loss, which presumably is largely skeletal, would amount to 50g calcium or approximately 4% of total skeletal calcium per year. . . . Since the subjects were all in negative calcium balance, there must have been loss of calcium from bone on the high protein diet."[4]

These are significant findings indicating that in a ten year period approximately 35% of skeletal calcium can be lost. Figures such as these demonstrate the inevitability of the development of osteoporosis not only in patients in the later years of life but also in patients in their 20s and 30s. We must remember that our dietary practices have changed dramatically since the 1960s — high protein fast-foods, convenience foods, preservatives, additives, meals-on-the-run — all are relatively recent innovations. A 60-year old man, his 40-year old son, and 20-year old grandson have all been exposed to this "new improved" life style for the same period of time. Consequently, each generation is equally as subject to the modern perils of excess protein and inadequate vegetable consumption, and each is losing alarming quantities of calcium.

Calcium loss from bones is normal on a short-term basis; this loss is compensated for by normal replacement. Bones continually lose and replace bone material. When the loss and replacement are balanced, normal bone physiology is maintained.

BLOOD CALCIUM, DIETARY CALCIUM, AND OSTEOPOROSIS

It is ironic that normal levels of calcium can exist in the blood while osteoporosis progresses unabated. Rarely do we find patients who have blood calcium levels below tolerable limits. We know that the body will maintain blood calcium levels at 9 to 10 mg/dl as a priority function. Calcium is necessary for proper muscle activity, blood coagulation, and other vital functions; consequently, the body will assure that this level is sustained. However, we cannot emphasize too strongly the inconsistency of osteoporotic degeneration of the bones taking place when the blood contains adequate levels of calcium. If there is a normal level of calcium in the blood and at the same time osteoporosis is taking its toll, one of two things must be true: either (1) the calcium level of the blood is not the primary factor in the development of osteoporosis, or (2) despite the level of calcium in the blood, this calcium is not usable by the body to prevent the disease.

In keeping with our assumption that the body never makes a mistake, we must conclude that the calcium consumed (usually in the form of dairy products) is not suitable for use by the body. If it were, conditions relating to calcium deficiency would not exist. The quality of serum calcium may not be high enough to replenish the bone matrix although it may be adequate to serve other purposes such as blood coagulation.

Although the body cannot use the calcium in dairy products to rebuild bones, deficiency of dietary calcium is not the cause of osteoporosis. McDougall writes: "Unprocessed vegetable foods contain sufficient calcium to meet the needs of adults and growing children. In fact, calcium deficiency caused by an insufficient amount of calcium in the diet is not known to occur in humans, even though most people in the world don't drink milk after weaning. . . ."[5] If sufficient calcium is available from daily diets, it becomes obvious that another factor is involved in the development of osteoporosis: too much protein or other acid-ash producing foods overwhelm the body's ability to neutralize and eliminate acid. In a sodium-deficient body, calcium is withdrawn from bones to be used to buffer the excess acid produced by continued excessive consumption of dietary protein.

The adage "milk is nature's best source of calcium" may be true, but further investigation demonstrates that it is not necessarily true for adult humans. The osteoporotic rate is higher in the people of countries where large quantities of milk is consumed than in the people of those countries where milk is not a staple of adults' everyday meals. Dietary calcium from cheese and other dairy products may enter the bloodstream resulting in a normal serum calcium reading, but it may not provide calcium of suitable quality for either buffering or replenishing bone matrix.

It is not possible to furnish the body enough calcium to prevent osteoporosis if protein consumption is too high. Dairy products, green leafy vegetables, and calcium supplements will not provide enough usable calcium for the body to overcome the ravages of excess protein. No matter what type of calcium is ingested — even organic calcium — it must be metabolized and personalized, and there is a delay between the time calcium is consumed and the time it becomes available for use.

PERSONALIZED CALCIUM

The concept of personalized calcium and other substances (even organs that are being transplanted) deals with the suitability of the newly acquired substance being of benefit to the host. Calcium in plants is utilized through their anabolic processes; however, when this calcium is taken into an individual's body, it must be acted upon by that individual's enzymes in order to be incorporated as a functioning ingredient. To accomplish this, the body must produce enzymes that will perform this function, as illustrated by the incident with the alfalfa-fed deer discussed earlier. The body produces enzymes on demand to serve a specific function.

OSTEOPOROSIS AND AGING

Although Guyton tells us ". . . calcium ion absorption is exactly controlled in relation to the need of the body for calcium,"[6] it is obvious from our discussion that high levels of calcium intake do not preclude the onset of osteoporosis. High levels of calcium in the blood do not assure continual redepositing of new bone matrix that is required to keep the bones strong and supportive.

Guyton recognizes the relationship between excess protein and deficient calcium but misses the crucial connection. He notes: ". . . many different diseases of protein metabolism can cause osteoporosis," and goes on to cite several causes, including: "old age, in which many of the protein anabolic functions are poor anyway so that bone matrix cannot be deposited satisfactorily."[7] From our discussions of the overall effect on the body of continued consumption of excess protein, we can postulate that these poor anabolic functions are the result of years of dietary abuse rather than of age.

If diminished bone matrix were strictly a function of aging, all peoples would experience a similar course of debilitation. However, studies show that the Bantus in Africa who consume only about 47 gm of protein and approximately 400 mg of calcium in their daily diet have virtually no osteoporosis. Their consumption of protein and acidifying foods is considerably less than that of the average American. In contrast, Eskimos who consume large quantities of both protein and calcium in their diets and who are physically very active have an exceptionally high rate of osteoporosis.[8] The most important factor that determines the availability of usable calcium to the body is the amount of acidifying foods in the diet, not the number of years lived. The primary impact of age would be the length of time the person had adhered to an excessively high protein diet. Once the body's neutralizing buffering systems have been overwhelmed by a long-term high-protein diet, even 47 gm of protein becomes excessive.

A study done by Anand and Linkswiler of the University of Wisconsin using nine young adult males as subjects quantifies the impact of excessive protein on the calcium balance of the body. The researchers wrote: "When the protein intake was 95 grams and 142 grams respectively, the mean calcium balance was -58 and -120 mg, and no subject was in calcium balance. Increasing the intake of fruits and vegetables by 50% had no beneficial effect on calcium balance."[9]

We can see by this study that the greater the amount of protein consumed, the greater the amount of calcium lost by the body. Calcium balance is maintained when the amount of calcium ingested equals the amount that is lost through urine or feces. A negative balance occurs when more calcium is eliminated than is consumed. In order for the body to eliminate more calcium than it takes in, a source other than diet must have been the origin of the eliminated calcium, and this source is the bones. When the body has been in a negative calcium balance situation over a period of time, even as little as 10 grams of protein per day may be more than the body can process without continuing to lose more calcium than is supplied.

THE RELATIONSHIP BETWEEN CALCIUM AND PHOSPHORUS

What is in acidifying foods that imposes such a great demand for calcium? The answer to this is "phosphorus." Phosphorus is a nonmetallic element not found in a free state, but is found in combination with alkalies as a phosphate. The body contains approximately 600-900 grams of phosphorus in various forms: 70-80% principally combined with calcium in bones and teeth, 10% in muscle, and 1% in nerve tissue.[10] Phosphorus, like protein, is a substance that our bodies need. Phosphorus is used in nerve transmission and in the production of ATP that stores energy in a form the body can readily use. However, again, it is necessary to maintain balance — too much of any element in the body, even a vitamin and mineral, causes reactions that may not be in the best interest of homeostasis and total body health. Too much of any one constituent can cause a functional deficiency of collateral components.

Calcium and phosphorus levels are regulated by Vitamin D and hormones of the parathyroid and thyroid glands. Calcium should be in equilibrium between the bloodstream and bones. When the blood calcium falls, the parathyroid will secrete a hormone that will stimulate osteoclastic activity which will release calcium and phosphorus from bone. The calcium is still "tied" to phosphorus even as it comes from the bone. However, the body certainly would not take calcium from the bone in order to extract the phosphorus that goes along with it — a person on a high protein diet already has too much phosphorus. Additional hormones secreted by the body will cause the phosphorus to be excreted by the kidneys, leaving available calcium for the body to use as a buffer or as serum calcium.

It bears repeating that it is not necessarily the amount of calcium in the diet that determines an adequate supply for the body. Rather, it is the quality of the dietary calcium and the extent of the demands for buffering placed on a diminishing alkaline reserve that determine if reserves are sufficient to perform the neutralizing functions required at any one time. The body establishes a relationship between the calcium and phosphorus that is stored principally in the bones. *A diet high in phosphorus is equivalent to a diet low in calcium.* The effects of the presence of excess amounts of phosphorus are the same as the effects of a calcium deficiency.

THE CALCIUM-PHOSPHORUS RATIO

The diet should contain foods that provide approximately two and one-half to three times as much calcium as phosphorus or the body will ultimately be stressed to maintain that homeostatic ratio. Guyton talks about the calcium in plasma and interstitial fluid as being 9-10 milligrams per deciliter (mg/dl), and of phosphorus being 3-4 mg/dl.[11] By taking the extremes of these two amounts, we can see that the ratio of calcium to phosphorus is between 2.5:1 and 3:l.

Milk is an excellent example of a high-calcium containing substance that is credited with providing us needed dietary calcium. However, in light of its calcium to phosphorus ratio, the validity of this cultural concept bears closer examination. Although in human milk the ratio of calcium to phosphorus and the presence of other elements in the milk are such that there is an overall alkalizing effect on infants, this is not equally true of cow's milk. The following table reveals a significant difference in both the calcium to phosphorus ratio and the protein content between human milk and cow's or goat's milk.

RATIO OF CALCIUM TO PHOSPHORUS IN MILK[12]

	Protein (mg)	Calcium (mg)	Phosphorus (mg)	Ratio
Human Milk	1.1	33	14	2.36:1
Cow's Milk	3.5	117	92	1.27:1
Goat's Milk	3.2	129	106	1.22:1

If we consider the calcium to phosphorus ratio (or the alkalizing to acidifying ratio) of mother's milk, it becomes apparent that our diet should contain a minimum of two times (or preferably, two and one-half times) as much calcium as phosphorus.

In addition to its less favorable phosphorus (phosphate) to calcium ratio, cow's milk has approximately three times as much protein as human milk. This is reflected in the total ash content of cow's milk being over three times that of human milk.[13] Increased acid places an even greater demand on the buffering systems which can require even more calcium. Since we know that the ash of protein has an acidifying effect on the body, it becomes apparent why cow's milk — pasteurized or not — can have a negative effect on the calcium balance and why the countries where people drink the greatest quantities of milk have the highest rate of bone fractures. These observations give credence to the premise that human consumption of cow's milk may contribute to the development of osteoporosis.

This interpretation of the effects of milk on physiology should not be construed as a condemnation of milk for infants. Milk is the staple that provides infants the nutrients they need for the rapid growth of their first years of development. Mother's milk is far superior to cow's milk, goat's milk, or formula preparations. However, milk is not recommended for adults. In addition to milk being a negative calcium source, adults do not tolerate milk as well as do infants. "After the age of four years, most people naturally lose the ability to digest the carbohydrate known as lactose found in milk, because they no longer synthesize the digestive enzyme, lactase, which lines the small intestine. This condition, known as lactose intolerance, results in symptoms of diarrhea, gas, and stomach cramps when lactose-containing dairy products are eaten."[14](McDougall)

Although there is calcium in milk, it is unsuitable for neutralizing the acidifying effect of the milk itself. Cow's milk has a preponderance of acidifying elements that produce an increased amount of acid which the body must neutralize.

THE EFFECTS OF PHOSPHORUS AND ACIDIFYING FOODS

Most sources of calcium, other than fruits and vegetables, contain large amounts of phosphorus, and we have established that a calcium to phosphorus ratio of at least 2:1 must be maintained throughout the body. We shall see how consuming calcium-rich foods that contain an equally high or higher level of phosphorus is self-defeating.

The beneficial ratio of calcium to phosphorus in the diet is illustrated in an experiment reported in Kamen's *Osteoporosis* [15] in which small dogs developed marked osteoporosis on a diet with a calcium-phosphorus ratio of 1:10. The osteoporosis was reversed when the ratio was reduced to 1:1. This research project demonstrates that no matter how much calcium is consumed, if phosphorus consumption is higher than calcium, and acid-ash producing foods put an additional drain on the resources of the buffering systems, calcium loss will result.

Phosphorus is absorbed into the blood more readily than is calcium. Guyton tells us: "Except for the portion of phosphate that is excreted in the feces in combination with calcium, almost all the dietary phosphate is absorbed into the blood from the gut and later excreted in the urine."[16] If phosphorus is absorbed more rapidly from the gut than calcium and then excreted from the kidney, there is a period of time when the phosphorus is in the blood, giving the blood a more acid reaction with which the body must deal. When sodium is no longer available from the alkaline reserve, calcium will be used in the initial buffering stages to neutralize the acid as the body seeks to maintain the required 7.4 pH of blood. The most readily available source of calcium in an alkaline deficient body is the bones. However, when the calcium is extracted from the bones, phosphorus is extracted with it which further complicates the situation.

Now with additional phosphorus in the blood, additional calcium is needed from the bones and, as we have seen, this calcium is accompanied by more phosphorus. Although the phosphorus can be eliminated through the kidneys, the demand for more calcium occurs while the phosphorus is in the bloodstream.

Kamen tells us: "A normal healthy body can utilize foods whether they are alkaline or acid. The blood acts as a buffer system to protect your normal pH. Fruits and vegetables in general are more alkaline because of their mineral content."[17] A "normal healthy body" is one in which an adequate alkaline reserve is present. However, we have seen in previous sections that there are limitations to sustaining the protective pH levels when some of the necessary counterparts become exhausted.

CALCIUM AND PROTEIN

We must understand that there is a difference between the acid formed in the body from protein-rich meats, grains, and dairy products, and the acid formed from carbohydrates such as fats, candies, and bakery products. The acid that is formed by meats and dairy products must be buffered before being eliminated through the kidneys — a process that can deplete the body's mineral reserves of sodium, potassium, and calcium. The acid that is produced by the metabolism of carbohydrates and fats (which are concentrated carbohydrates) is carbonic acid that can be eliminated through the lungs and cause no drain on the mineral reserves. This difference is important; the acid that is produced from carbohydrates and fats is similar to the acid that is produced in exercise. These acids, in and of themselves, do not drain the body's mineral reserves; however, if an already high acid level produced by a diet of excess meats, grains and carbohydrates is compounded by the acid produced by regular, vigorous exercise, the problems associated with alkaline reserve depletion are exacerbated. As we have seen, the only solution to this chronic degenerative disease-producing situation is to reduce the consumption of acid-ash producing foods and increase the consumption of fruits and vegetables.

Guyton illustrates the difference between the amount of calcium in bone and the amount in extracellular fluid: "Bone contains such great amount of calcium in comparison with the total amount in all the extracellular fluids (about 1000 times as much) that even when parathyroid hormone causes a great rise in calcium concentration in the fluids, it is impossible to discern any immediate effect on the bones."[18] He also points out that 41% of the calcium in plasma and interstitial fluid is hooked to protein, 9% is diffusible but un-ionized, and 50% is an ionic calcium.[19]

The calcium that is hooked to its partner in an ionic bond may not be as usable by the body even though it is ionizable. Calcium chloride could be seen as an example of calcium that is not usable even though it is ionized. The bond unifying this compound could be too strong to be broken by the body's covalent enzymatic system. Even if calcium chloride could be ionized into calcium ions and chloride ions, the strong attraction for the two remains. In our discussion of the replacement capabilities of different elements (Chapter Nine), we show the ranking of elements in accordance with their ability to gain or lose electrons as given in the activity, or electromotive, series. In order for the calcium to be replaced by another substance in the electromotive series, a substance higher in the series than calcium must be used. The only two elements that qualify are lithium and potassium. (Lithium is used as a drug in the treatment of some mental illnesses and can be toxic to the body, and potassium is an integral part of the phosphate buffer system.) Since calcium and hydrogen are both positive ions, it may appear that the hydrogen ion should be able to replace the calcium ion in calcium chloride leaving hydrogen chloride. However, hydrogen is lower than calcium in the electromotive series which means it is less active than calcium. The calcium could replace the hydrogen in hydrogen chloride to form calcium chloride, but hydrogen cannot replace calcium.

In order for calcium to be available for the body to use, it must be hooked to a substance that the body can process in its normal metabolic route. When the partner substance is metabolized, calcium is available for other uses. However, calcium in the body that is hooked to an ionic substance cannot be released by enzymatic action. Calcium that is determined to be ionic through laboratory analysis may have been "killed" in the testing process and may merely appear to be ionic. If the calcium is from a metabolized substance, such as calcium caseinate, the calcium is available to the body to be used either as a buffer or in the metabolic process. A good example of this is the calcium that is attached to protein — the body can metabolize and utilize this calcium.

Yet, generally calcium that is attached to protein is accompanied by phosphorus. If the phosphorus is in greater amounts than the calcium, the calcium yields a negative reward. As infants, the only place that we can get calcium is in calcium caseinate — a protein found originally in mother's milk. Again we see that calcium is attached to a protein molecule. The body digests the protein molecule leaving the calcium to be used by the body wherever it is needed. As adults, our main source of calcium should be fruits and vegetables that have calcium in combination with organic acids. Metabolism of the organic acid will leave free calcium available for the body to use as a buffering agent and to replenish the bone matrix to normal physiological levels.

Calcium sometimes appears as an extra precipitate in the rib cartilage; it is not supposed to be there — especially in patients who have osteoporosis and are losing calcium from the bones. Some calcium gets into the blood to give us a normal reading of the calcium level, but it is unable to perform the normal buffering function. Once calcium that is unsuitable for normal physiological function gets into the blood, it must be disposed of and the cartilage can serve as a storage area until it can be reabsorbed and eliminated. This illustrates how normal blood calcium levels can be found although the patient is experiencing active osteoporosis.

CALCIUM SUPPLEMENTS

It is important to recall that individual elements, vitamins, or minerals are not substitutes for whole foods and a balanced diet. Our dietary regimen should consist of whole foods that contain all of the substances that the body needs. When complete foods are supplied, the body will use the individual vitamins, minerals, and nutrients needed to maintain homeostasis without being burdened by the additional stress of dealing with partial or fabricated foods. Supplementation can be temporarily therapeutic for patients whose physical conditions are extreme, however, it should be used strictly on a short-term basis.

One of the factors associated with supplements that negates their effectiveness is that the substances from which they are made are "dead." That is, supplements are produced from substances that may have been living at one time but these substances have been processed to the point that their vitality has been eliminated. It is essential that we consume foods that have retained their vitality, or living quality.

The following recipe describes a method of preparing a calcium supplement that retains the vitality of the ingredients and provides "living" covalent calcium that the body can assimilate and use. "Lemon Egg" (also known as "Egg Calcium") can be made inexpensively by patients and can bolster the depleted calcium supply without placing an additional burden on the body's delicate balance. However, this preparation is extremely powerful and patients should be cautioned to limit their daily consumption to only ONE TEASPOONFUL per day. For those whose bodies are not accustomed to consuming sufficient amounts of usable calcium, violation of this word of caution will almost certainly lead to leg cramps.

LEMON EGG

Carefully fill a wide-mouth fruit jar with clean, whole, uncracked eggs. Cover the eggs with *freshly squeezed*, strained lemon juice. Cover the jar loosely and place in the refrigerator. Gently agitate the jar a few times during the day. Bubbles will appear around the eggs. After approximately 48 hours, when the bubbling has stopped, remove the eggs from the jar, being careful not to break them. Replace the lid tightly and shake the mixture well.

The shells of the eggs are softened by the chemical action of the citric acid of the lemon which allows the calcium to combine with the lemon juice as calcium citrate. If the eggs are left in the mixture for more than 48 hours, the mixture will begin to thicken and the eggs will begin to absorb more of the lemon taste. Should an egg be broken while it is in the liquid or being removed, the mixture will still be usable, however, its shelf-life will be greatly reduced.

The calcium in the lemon egg mixture is a living substance; neither the eggs nor the lemon have been exposed to heat above a normal living temperature, and the eggs are still usable. The mixture should not be heated since heat destroys the vitality of any living material.

It is not necessary to increase the daily quantity of Lemon Egg in order to reap sustained benefits. Again, a reminder for those patients who act on the premise "if a little bit is good for you, a lot must be better"; they should be cautioned that more than ONE TEASPOONFUL of egg calcium a day will cause muscle cramps. This may not happen immediately, however, within a few weeks the patient will begin to experience attention-getting cramps in muscles. If an over-infusion of calcium into the system causes muscle cramps, the patient should discontinue the egg calcium for a week and then reinstate the dosage of ONE TEASPOONFUL OR LESS each day.

Of at least equal importance to the amount of egg calcium taken each day is the other food that is included in the daily diet along with this potent usable calcium supplement. It is very important to EXCLUDE ALL MILK AND CHEESE from the diet of a patient who is taking egg calcium.

Patients who regularly consume milk, cheese, and other dairy products have already overloaded their bodies with calcium that cannot be used and they have not had an opportunity to rid themselves of this inorganic substance. Since the calcium from the egg shells is readily available, the body begins to use this needed mineral. However, when egg calcium is taken along with milk or cheese, a means of disposing of the inappropriate calcium from the milk and other dairy products must be found. As usable, organic calcium goes into the blood stream, the inorganic calcium may cause kidney stones or diseases associated with too much calcium even though there is not enough usable calcium. Patients must stop consuming dairy products when they begin to add covalent calcium of the lemon egg mixture to their daily diets.

It is imperative that patients understand that egg calcium should be a source of calcium only on a short-term basis. The calcium provided in this mixture is highly concentrated. Usually one month of supplementation with lemon egg will be adequate to bridge the transition period between the time additional fruits and vegetables are introduced into the diet and the time the body can fully utilize the calcium they provide. Over the long-term, fruits and vegetables provide the balance of nutrients — including calcium — that nature intended. For example, in fruits and vegetables, the magnesium to calcium ratio is adequately balanced along with many other trace minerals.

When the level of organic calcium in the diet is increased, this calcium may not be used immediately by the body. We indicate throughout these chapters that nothing in the body happens in isolation — ancillary factors are always involved when any stimulus is introduced into the body. For example, vitamin D, a parathyroid hormone, and other components that work in tandem with calcium are not increased in equal proportions to the calcium of lemon egg. Consequently, when the additional calcium is taken into the body, all of the calcium may not be immediately available for use. If there is not an equal increase of the substances that are necessary for the calcium to be used, the function of the calcium will be diminished and symptoms of a calcium deficiency will appear. As additional usable calcium is made available, the affected systems of the body will gradually adjust to the improved calcium level, the calcium will be assimilated for use in its many functions, and the calcium in the bones will again be replenished.

By understanding the all-encompassing role excess protein plays in the body, we can see that a deficiency of calcium is not the culprit in osteoporosis — acidifying foods prevent calcium from remaining in the bones to keep them strong and durable. Reports of patients with osteoporosis whose bones break with little or no provocation at the age of 55 or above have been common for years. We are now seeing patients much younger than 55 who are experiencing these same problems. In my clinical experience, I have seen many farmers who consume large amounts of milk who have developed osteoporosis as well as calcium in the rib cartilage. Cases such as these would indicate that the body is stupid. However, the body's innate intelligence is far greater than man can ever hope to achieve. The body does everything for a reason. It is far better for the calcium concentration of bones to be diminished than for the body to suffer the consequences of life-threatening acid accumulation.

9

CHEMICAL REACTIONS IN THE BODY

Throughout this book we talk about how the body reacts to a variety of stimuli, particularly foods. We point out how our sodium supply can be depleted although there is sodium chloride in most of our food, and we note how nutritional deficiencies can develop even though our diets are supplemented with vitamins, minerals, and, perhaps, enzymes. A brief survey of the role of chemical reactions in the body should help to clarify some of these apparent paradoxes and reinforce our assertion that only whole foods supply the covalently bonded minerals the body requires to maintain an environment that promotes correct pH, homeostasis, and health.

REPLACEMENT REACTIONS

Chemical reactions may involve decomposition and composition in which one substance is broken apart and another is built; however, most of the chemical reactions pertinent to the concepts concerning pH presented here involve replacement reactions in which one element takes the place of another.

All non-nuclear chemical reactions are based on the ability of electrons to move. It is this movement of electrons that ties inorganic (or general) chemistry to biochemistry. An understanding of the factors involved in the movement of the electrons of elements leads to a better understanding of how the food we eat impacts physiology.

We stated in Chapter Three that oxidation is the process of combining a substance with oxygen to produce heat or energy. All food is oxidized after it is eaten but not in the same way as a piece of wood is oxidized by burning. Burning is a rapid oxidation process that creates a great deal of heat, and, although all oxidation produces a certain amount of heat, reactions inside the body must take place at 98.6 degrees Fahrenheit and must proceed at a relatively slow pace. Biological oxidation does not involve the direct addition of oxygen to carbon to form carbon dioxide; it involves the removal of hydrogen, or, simply, the removal of electrons. As we shall see later in this chapter, this process is carried out by the action of very specialized enzymes.

Although an in-depth look at chemical principles is beyond the scope of this book, a brief review of some of the basic terms may be helpful in clarifying the concepts associated with our discussion.

You will recall that an *atom* is the smallest particle of an element that can take part in a chemical reaction. It is electrically neutral, having equal numbers of protons (+) and electrons (-). In general, there are only three ways an atom can undergo change: it can (1) lose electrons, (2) gain electrons, or (3) share electrons. Whether atoms gain or lose electrons is determined by which process involves the least effort in the existing environment.

A *molecule* is the smallest part of a chemical substance that can exist independently — it consists of one or more atoms.

Electrons are negatively charged particles found in atoms; and *protons* are their positively charged counterparts. The addition of electrons to an atom increases negativity, the loss of electrons increases positivity. It is the transference of electrons that govern all non-nuclear chemical reactions.

An *ion* is an atom or group of atoms that has gained or lost one or more electrons, thereby becoming electrostatically charged.[1]

Chemical reactions occur in response to an inherent tendency in all substances to reach equilibrium — balance. When there is more energy in one substance than in another, this natural equilibrium-seeking tendency dominates. When an imbalance exists, equilibrium is re-established by the movement of electrons in a chemical reaction known as an oxidation-reduction reaction. Substances that gain electrons undergo reduction — substances that lose electrons are oxidized.[2] The tendency toward the movement of electrons has been calculated and relative values for the different elements have been set. The potential of an element's electrons to move is expressed as the oxidation-reduction potential, or simply, as the *oxidation potential.*[3]

The *ionization potential* is the ability of an atom to become an ion, (gain or lose electrons, become electrically imbalanced: atom → ion). The *electrode potential* is the ability of an ion to become an atom, (gain or lose electrons, become electrically balanced: ion → atom). Elements that are of high potential in one category (ionization or electrode) will be low in the other. But a comparison of ionization potential and electrode potential must be made on the basis of their position in their respective series, not on the number assigned since the measurements are made under different conditions.[4]

Metallic elements are ranked according to the ease with which they give up electrons — their oxidative potential. Using this ranking, an activity series, or electromotive force series, has been developed to show the decreasing order of oxidative potential. The abbreviated list that follows includes only the more common elements, their places in the activity series, and the electrode potential in volts of each.

This list shows elements in descending order of electron-losing ability with those at the top being more active and better able to lose electrons easily. The values assigned are important to our discussion since they offer a more vivid picture of the relative ease with which atoms acquire or release electrons, and nature (like man) ordinarily follows the course that requires the least amount of effort.

ACTIVITY SERIES[5]

Lithium	+3.02
Potassium	+2.92
Calcium	+2.87
Sodium	+2.71
Magnesium	+2.34
Aluminum	+1.67
Zinc	+0.76
Tin	+0.14
Lead	+0.13
Hydrogen	0.00
Copper	-0.34
Mercury	-0.80
Silver	-0.80
Gold	-0.68

The oxidative potential of hydrogen, listed as 0.00 electrode potential in volts, is the reference point for the activity series. The higher the electrode potential, the greater the tendency to lose electrons; the lower the electrode potential the more firmly fixed the electrons. Potassium, calcium, and sodium (elements of great activity) rank high on this list. These metals are so active that they will displace hydrogen from cold water. When pure sodium is dropped into water, the hydrogen replacement is so intense that a vigorous reaction occurs. Farther down the list is a group of metals including magnesium, aluminum, and zinc that are not as active but are still able to displace hydrogen from steam. Metals such as tin and lead that will displace hydrogen from acids are even farther down the list, just above hydrogen.[6]

This series is not only a measure of the elements' reactivity with water, steam, and acid, but also of their reactivity with each other. In an acid medium, potassium will replace calcium or sodium in a reaction because potassium is more active than either of the other two. Sodium cannot replace potassium; elements can be replaced only by those higher in the activity series. However, the action of calcium, under certain conditions, would appear to invalidate this tenet as its ionization potential does not remain constant.

Ionization should not be confused with dissolution. Ionization of an atom changes the number of electrons of an atom while dissolution changes the physical characteristics of a compound. As you will recall from basic chemistry, the compound NaCl does not contain molecules except at very high temperatures; sodium chloride is composed of two elements containing atoms.[7] If a teaspoon of table salt is placed in a beaker of water, the salt will dissolve and be visually indistinguishable from the water. However, the salt is still apparent to taste — it has dissolved in water but has retained its own identity. If the water is boiled away, the same NaCl will remain in the same crystalline structure it had before being dissolved. Hydrogen cannot replace sodium ions in NaCl or in any other compound.

In considering the valence, or degree of combining power, of the various elements, it might be assumed that since both hydrogen and sodium have a +1 charge the two elements have the same replacement potential. However, sodium is high on the activity chart and hydrogen is low, therefore hydrogen cannot replace sodium in chemical reactions. Sodium will replace hydrogen UNLESS the sodium is connected to another element by a strong electrovalent bond as in the case of sodium chloride. This bond may be stronger than the tendency of sodium to replace hydrogen; it is the strength of this bond that accounts for the body's inability to use the sodium of table salt to replenish the alkaline reserve.[8] In addition, electrovalent bonds are always stronger than covalent bonds.[9] The body is designed to function with covalent bonds and cannot effectively split ionic bonds or overcome the powerful attraction each ion has for its partner. Even after the sodium chloride becomes 100% ionized in water, the powerful attraction between the sodium and chloride still exists.

It is valid to argue that the body contains substances that will replace sodium. However, in order to accomplish this, the replacing elements must be higher than sodium on the activity series, i.e., calcium, potassium, and lithium. As the body becomes deficient in sodium, it will offset this deficiency with calcium.

Lithium is even higher on the activity series than are sodium, calcium, or potassium and has been used in the treatment of specific emotional disorders. Lithium can replace any or all of these elements in a chemical reaction, but just a slight amount becomes highly toxic to the body. This is an example of a successful laboratory reaction proving to be unsuccessful biochemically.

THE SIGNIFICANCE OF REPLACEMENT

By relating some of these general chemistry facts to biochemistry, we can illustrate just how significant they are. We know that energy must be generated in the form of ATP if the body is to continue to function and that oxygen is needed for efficient production of ATP. The movement of hydrogen ions and electrons with the aid of enzymes is vital to this process. The body splits O_2 into two oxygen radicals, each of which has a tremendous attraction for hydrogen ions; when the hydrogen and oxygen unite, water is formed. There is always an abundance of hydrogen ions since normal cellular metabolism produces carbonic acid (H_2CO_3). However, when the oxygen supply to the cell is diminished, sufficient quantities of oxygen ions are not available to combine with the hydrogen ions. At the same time, hydrogen ions are being produced by other sources (such as acid-ash producing foods) and their numbers increase. The resulting excess of hydrogen ions compounds the problem of maintaining sufficient oxygen ions for ATP production.

As more meat is consumed, more acid is produced and more hydrogen ions are generated. However, at the same time, the high acid concentration causes the blood to become more acid which diminishes its oxygen carrying ability. With less oxygen available, cellular glycolysis and the production of ATP must shift from an aerobic state to an anaerobic state which (as noted in Chapter Three) results in a ten-fold decrease in efficiency. Concurrently, less oxygen is available to split into oxygen ions that can combine with the hydrogen ions to form water. We can see that as the hydrogen ion concentration increases, the body's ability to deal with this situation is impaired.

THE REVERSAL OF CALCIUM AND POTASSIUM

Calcium exhibits a characteristic that is unique among the more common elements: the ionization potential of calcium changes according to whether it is in an acid or alkaline environment, and this change affects the calcium's activity in chemical reactions. Although, as yet, physiologists have been unable to explain this phenomenon, I submit the following evidence, observations, and resulting hypothesis for consideration.

1. The ionization potential of calcium changes from 2.87 in an acid medium to 3.02 in an alkaline medium.[10]

2. The change in the environment from acid to alkaline could be a primary factor that causes calcium to release electrons more easily.

3. As calcium becomes more active than potassium, the following reactions could occur:

    a. The calcium ions form a stronger bond with non-metals rendering them more stable in precipitated form and causing them to be deposited in joints producing pain and stiffness (arthritis).

b. Calcium contributes more electrons than potassium to non-metal substances which could cause a deficiency of calcium for all other reactions and create an elevated serum potassium concurrently with advanced osteoporosis. (Clinical observations as evidenced by x-rays and blood analysis.)

As the intracellular and extracellular environments become alkaline due to the accumulation of ammonia brought about by processing excess protein, patients may experience temporary or long-term symptoms.

a. Some patients break out in hives or experience other allergic reactions immediately after consuming citrus fruits or tomato juice. (More acid is added to a body that is already metabolically over-acidic. Although the additional citric acid is organic and will leave an alkaline ash, this new substance has not yet been metabolized to provide the beneficial effects.)

b. These same patients, or those who do not have an immediate allergic reaction, may experience morning stiffness in joints which indicates an arthritic tendency.

As protein consumption continues to raise the acid level of the body, the intracellular fluids and, to a lesser degree, extracellular fluids become congested with ammonia. Ammonia, being an alkaline substance, tends to raise the alkalinity of the cell. In an alkaline medium, the electrode potential of calcium changes from +2.87 to +3.02. When the alkalinity of the cell is raised, the active calcium that is normally on the cell membrane is drawn into the cell. Potassium moves from the inside of the cell to the outside in order to maintain a normal osmotic and electric balance. This movement of potassium to the outside of the cell is only in response to the calcium becoming more active and moving inside the cell in order to maintain proper osmolarity and polarity. Sodium's position under these circumstances remains constant — it remains extracellular. However, by the time ammonia has begun to accumulate intracellularly, a sodium deficiency is already evident. This phenomenon would explain the apparent contradictions of a patient simultaneously expressing osteoporosis, elevated serum potassium, stiffness and joint pain.

Hypothesis: Reversal of calcium and potassium occurs in an alkaline medium created by ammonia. Although to date this premise has not been substantiated by laboratory analysis, I believe that research into the pH of body fluids that include excess ammonia would reveal data that would either confirm or refute this hypothesis and have a significant impact on biochemistry. I would welcome such data.

SUPPLEMENTATION

If the doctor determines through analysis that there is a deficiency of particular substances, such as vitamins or minerals, and has the patient supplement those particular substances, the patient generally experiences immediate relief. However, the supplementation can send false signals to the body that will lead to a deficiency of other vitamins and minerals.

Any fragments of food, including vitamin and mineral supplements, have a stimulatory effect on the body. If a patient is deficient in a particular vitamin and he takes supplements of that vitamin in tablet form, he should understand that the quantities of supplements in that tablet are completely arbitrary and very likely disproportionate to what his body needs. If he feels better after taking the vitamin, it is due to the stimulatory effect on his body, not to an improvement in overall health. All vitamins work together; supplementing a single vitamin disturbs the balance thereby creating a deficiency of all other vitamins that are necessary for that vitamin or the system to operate properly.

If the vitamin does satisfy a deficiency, the proportions will almost certainly be wrong with respect to all of the other vitamins, thus upsetting the synergy of the entire system. Each vitamin or mineral represents a very complex substance that requires enzymes, coenzymes and other substances in order to function at maximum efficiency. No one has just a vitamin deficiency, although he may have a system deficiency.

Any supplementation must be viewed as being strictly a temporary measure to be employed only while the total dietary picture is gradually improved. It is *impossible* to make a poor diet into a good diet by supplementation. We need to increase the intake of whole foods and decrease the amount of food fragments, including vitamin and mineral supplements, if we are to achieve balance.

Only those vitamins and minerals that have been prepared as closely as possible to natural concentration and composition should be recommended. The more concentrated the vitamin, the more stimulatory it becomes. Concentrated and refined supplementation products are never equal to food as found in nature — any living system is always greater than the sum of its parts.

FRAGMENTED FOOD

Fragmented food — food that has been refined, processed, or synthesized — requires the same digestive processes as whole food. Refined foods are devoid of life, consequently, they are devoid of enzymes. In order to digest fragmented, lifeless food, the body must first make enzymes from previously stored material. The body can cope occasionally with fragmented refined foods that provide only "empty calories." However, when these foods consistently make up a major portion of the diet, eventually the reserves, including digestive enzymes, needed to process the incomplete foods will be depleted.

Enzymes from food provide the vitality the body needs to carry on life. Without the vitality provided by raw, whole, living, constructive foods, the body cannot *properly* replenish and rebuild the cells that are the elemental structures of our physical being.

When fresh, raw fruits and vegetables are eaten, all of the vitamins, minerals, and enzymes needed to process that food are consumed. The body needs only to rearrange the materials to digest it completely and easily. Whole foods such as fruits and vegetables have the added advantage of making a small deposit to the alkaline reserve — they never make a withdrawal.

A slice of white bread, on the other hand, is virtually devoid of enzymes and minerals. The argument could be made that supplements can compensate for this. Unfortunately, even though food supplements get into the body under the guise of food, they will not make up for the deficiency. For example, when the body tries to utilize a calcium supplement, the calcium concentration is so high that the enzymes, coenzymes, and cofactors needed to utilize the calcium are now deficient by comparison. As a result, the system responds as it would if there were a deficiency of calcium. Although there is no deficiency, the symptoms are the same as if there were.

At the turn of this century, D.D. Palmer, the founder of chiropractic, saw little need to dwell on the nutritional aspects of health, and with good reason. At that time, foods were considerably more "natural" than they are today. Processing, refining, and synthesizing food had not yet appeared on the scene, and meat was more of a delicacy for special occasions than standard daily fare. Our affluent society, with instant meals, prepared foods and fast-food restaurants, removes a great deal of drudgery from our lives, but we are paying more than we realize in terms of health as a result of the rapidly diminishing quality of food that is accepted as standard by the general public.

The way the body responds to fragments of food illustrates the fact that everything in the body works together to achieve homeostasis. Parts of food are suitable only as a short-term emergency treatment — an interim measure that can be detrimental if continued over long periods of time. Supplementation may change symptoms but will not make the patient more healthy; only by improving eating and life style habits can he accomplish that.

ENZYMES — CONSUMED AND PRODUCED

General chemistry and biochemistry are often viewed as separate studies, however, it is clear that they are interrelated. Chemical reactions are integral parts of physiological processes; minute chemical functions involving ions, electrons, elements, and enzymes can have far-reaching effects on the entire physical system. However, a given laboratory-produced reaction cannot be unquestionably extrapolated to living systems. Laboratory reactions tend to be associated with high heat which destroys the key to all living systems — living enzymes.

Enzymes are produced by living plants and animals. Enzymes cause changes in other substances without being changed themselves — enzymes act as catalysts. In living plants, enzymes serve a metabolic function of building new tissue. Enzymes can be destroyed by high temperatures but they are rendered inert by low temperatures. Fruit that has been refrigerated is an excellent example of a living plant containing inactive enzymes. A peach bought at the supermarket may appear to be ripe; however, if the peach has been kept at low temperatures, it will be hard and tasteless or bitter. After it has been warmed to room temperature for 24 to 48 hours, it will be softer and more tasty — the enzymes contained in the peach have resumed the ripening and maturing process.

Thousands of enzymes have been identified as the precipitating factors in the many chemical reactions of the body, yet there are still other reactions for which enzymes have not been identified. Dr. Edward Howell, in his book *Enzyme Nutrition*[11], writes: "Hundreds of metabolic enzymes are necessary to carry on the work of the body — to repair damage and decay, and heal diseases."

Enzymes are present in natural whole foods, and enzymes are secreted within the body for the digestion of foods. Dr. Howell uses the terms "exogenous food enzymes" that are present in living food before it has been cooked, and "endogenous (internal) enzymes with the enzyme reinforcements needed to check the disease-making process."[12] The enzymes in whole food act to complete the development and maturing of the food material. If a fruit is picked before it has ripened, enzymes will cause the ripening process to continue. If the fruit is not otherwise destroyed or cooked, the ripening process continues until the fruit disintegrates. However, if the food is eaten, heat of the body stimulates the enzymes to faster action and these enzymes continue to mature and ripen the food. When this takes place inside the body, the process is termed digestion. The function of the enzymes in the fruit or plant does not change just because the enzyme is in the stomach.

Enzymes in food help to begin the digestive process in the stomach. Living enzymes in the food we eat initiate the digestion of that food while it is in the stomach. Much of the natural digestion of the food we eat should take place in the stomach through the continued ripening and maturing process brought about by the enzymes. Raw fruits and vegetables contain all of the enzymes necessary to digest (ripen) their constituent parts — carbohydrates, proteins, and fats — almost completely. During this initial digestion stage, the pH of the stomach conforms to that required for the substance being digested. The pH remains high while carbohydrates are being digested, and it becomes lower for digestion of proteins and fats. For example, in the digestion of a potato that has 2% protein, the pH will remain high while the starch is digested and drop to the appropriate acidity to digest the small amount of protein.

Those portions of carbohydrates, proteins, and fats that are not completely digested by their own enzymes pass into the duodenum. Here an evaluation is made — without thought — of the chemical structure of the substance and the enzymes of the pancreas continue the job of digesting the food. These pancreatic enzymes are acting as a backup or finishing touch to the natural digestion initiated by the enzymes in whole, uncooked foods.

It is understandable that there are misconceptions about the function of enzymes, the difference between "consumed" and "produced" enzymes, and the effect they have on one another.

My research and experience indicate that our bodies use only substances (both those produced internally and those that are ingested) that are highly personalized. If we were to inject some of Patient A's pepsin into Patient B, I am convinced that B would not be able to utilize this enzyme until it had been rearranged to suit his personal physiological structure. By the same token, if a comparatively simple substance such as calcium were transferred from A to B, the calcium would need to be rearranged and adapted to make it specific to B. Patient B might be able to use A's calcium, but only after it had been personalized.

Since the body produces enzymes that will digest the type of food an individual is accustomed to eating, changes in the diet should be made carefully. The body must have time to adapt during a diet change before it can produce an enzyme it hasn't used or needed for a long time — if ever. This delay in adaptation was illustrated by the story of snowbound deer that starved to death although they had eaten their fill of air-dropped alfalfa hay — their systems could not generate the specific enzymes to digest the "foreign" substances in time to keep them from starving to death.

Much of the food available in supermarkets has been refined or processed and contains no enzymes. When refined foods are eaten, the body must make the needed digestive enzymes "from scratch." This, of course, adds another stress factor that makes the body work harder than should be necessary. Whole natural foods, on the other hand, provide enzyme building blocks that the body can easily use.

The important thing to realize is that the body must have enzymes in order for the digestive process to occur. These enzymes can come either from external sources in raw foods or from internal sources such as the pancreas. If enzymes from foods are not available, additional pancreatic enzymes are required which places additional stress on the body. Recall that the pH of the pancreatic secretion is 8.00 - 8.30 — quite alkaline as compared with that of the stomach. Pancreatic enzymes operate in a rather narrow pH range. In a process analogous to that of the diminishing sodium supply of the buffering system, over-dependence on internally generated pancreatic enzymes can result in loss of overall vitality and increased susceptibility to chronic degenerative disease. Just as it is vital that we replenish our sodium supply by eating fruits and vegetables, it is imperative that we reinforce our enzyme supply by making sure raw fruits and vegetables are included in our daily diet.

COOKING AFFECTS THE COMPONENTS OF FOOD

Enzymes are destroyed by heat. Any temperature above 130 degrees Fahrenheit will inactivate enzymes. Cooking destroys the enzymes present in food thereby reducing the level of vitality of cooked food to less than that of the body. As a result, the body is required to use some of its own vitality to impart energy to the food.

The effect of cooked food on living animals was demonstrated by a research project conducted over a period of five years using more than 100 cats as subjects.[13] Some of the cats were kept on a diet of natural, raw protein food while others were fed cooked foods such as pasteurized milk, cooked eggs, and boiled or roasted meat. The natural-food group thrived, bred and produced several generations of normal kittens. The cats that were fed cooked protein developed diseases similar to those seen in man — pyorrhea, liver disease, and nervous system damage. In addition, the kittens of the first generation of the cooked-food group were stunted and unable to reproduce. However, the findings after the project had ended were equally as startling. The researchers found that the soil that had been fertilized by the cats of the cooked-food group would not support new plant life — even weeds!

Although the metabolism and physiology of cats and humans are distinctly different, this experiment clearly illustrates that foods should be eaten in the most natural state possible — raw fruits and vegetables are preferable since cooking severely alters food. For example, cold-processed oil, made from seeds or grain, that has not been heated above 130 degrees in the extraction process contains enzymes that are still viable and will supply materials the body can use. Cooking with cold-processed oil, however, would defeat the purpose of the cold-processing since heat destroys the enzymes. Clinical research has substantiated the claim that when raw foods make up approximately 30% of the diet, the body will be supplied with the living qualities it needs.

Cooking affects other constituents of food in addition to enzymes, such as calcium in pasteurized milk. Pasteurizing milk renders the calcium it contains less available for living functions. This was illustrated when calves that had been fed pasteurized milk died after two months on this natural diet of milk made unnatural by pasteurization.[14] The calcium may assume a more electrovalent type bond that inhibits it from serving the function of personalized calcium required for replenishing bones or neutralizing acids. It is ironic that the more milk that is consumed, the more opportunity there is for osteoporosis to develop. This can be explained by understanding that for man's digestive system, there are more acidifying elements than alkalizing elements in cow's milk. Consequently, the more milk that is consumed, the more sodium is required to satisfy the acidifying effect the milk has on the body. If the diet is such that excessive amounts of acid-ash producing foods are eaten, including milk, covalent sodium will not be available to replenish the sodium reserves. These reserves will ultimately be depleted, and calcium (also high in the activity series) will be required to neutralize the excess acid that has been produced by the consumption and degradation of protein. Raw milk may afford more usable calcium than pasteurized milk, but it still retains the acidifying properties. The heat of pasteurization (as with other forms of cooking) converts an unsatisfactory food into an undesirable substance.

Modern man has cooked and killed the very substances that initiate natural digestion in the stomach. Our diets consist predominantly of food that no longer contains viable, usable, beneficial enzymes. Research reports tell us that digestion does not take place in the stomach, however, this research has been conducted using food that has been cooked. The results of the research under these circumstances is correct — the enzymes in cooked food have been rendered useless and unable to begin digestion. Since digestion of cooked food cannot take place in the stomach, the backup system of pancreatic enzymes then becomes the paramount and primary digestive system. As we have seen with other systems of the body, adaptive measures can be handled for a time but prolonged accommodation to deficiencies takes its toll on health.

ENZYME INHIBITORS

Periodically we hear of archaeologists unearthing grains and seeds that have been entombed for hundreds of years. Grains and seeds are viable entities that can lie dormant for long periods then germinate when moisture and temperature conditions are right. Until conditions are favorable, enzyme inhibitors in seeds prevent enzymatic action that begins the sprouting process. It is these inhibitors that cause digestive distress if the seeds and grains are eaten while the inhibitors prevail. Cooking dormant seeds and grains destroys the enzyme inhibitors but it also destroys the enzymes. Under conditions that allow seeds or grains to germinate, enzymes are released that inactivate the enzyme inhibitors. In the first hours of germination, enzymes become active and enzyme inhibitors are negated.

Modern agricultural practices allow for faster, more extensive and efficient methods of collecting crops from the field. Grains are now removed from the stalk immediately after cutting. This practice is more economical than former methods, but a vital transitional period is eliminated. In the past, grain remained on the stalk in the field after cutting. During this time, the grain was exposed to moisture and sun which allowed enzymes to be released and produced and the germination process to begin. Current practices deliver mature but dormant grains to food processors to be transformed into virtually enzyme-free products. Enzymes may be added to consumer products artificially, which is helpful in the manufacturing of bread and bakery products, but the added enzymes are of little or no benefit to the person who eats the food.[15]

PRIORITIES OF DIGESTION

The type of food that goes into the stomach determines how the body responds. If you eat only starches at a meal, the pH of the stomach will stay above 5. If you eat protein and starch food (such as wheat), the pH of the stomach will remain high while the carbohydrates are being digested, and the acidity will then be increased to digest the protein. When protein and starch are included in one food, the body can deal with the different properties in order of dominance. However, when the protein and starch are eaten together in two separate foods — such as steak and potatoes — the body is still faced with digesting the dominant substance but the dominance changes from protein to starch and back to protein again as dominance in terms of volume of the two is altered. Under these conditions, the digestive functions fluctuate in a manner that is Necessary but not Natural. On the other hand, if vegetables are eaten with either the potato or the protein, the body will first take care of the dominant starch or protein and then digest the vegetables. Since raw vegetables are high in water content and enzymes, they usually put no extreme stress on the digestion process.

ENZYME SUPPLEMENTS

We have been led to believe that little digestion takes place in the stomach because very few enzymes are secreted there. However, it is in the stomach that the enzymes contained in the food we eat can do their job of continuing to ripen or break down food fibers.

Many supplemental enzyme products are animal pancreatic extracts that are coated to allow the tablet to pass through the stomach to the small intestine. These tablets supplement the patient's pancreatic enzymes, but they do not enhance the process that should take place in the stomach. Enzymes that are part of raw foods begin the digestive process in the mouth and continue in the stomach without inflicting additional burdens on the internal enzymatic system.

The body was designed to run on good, wholesome food which has been grown in rich, vital soil. The body is able to assimilate and utilize the specific nutrients it needs from well-grown food. However, since most patients have unknowingly been diminishing their pancreatic enzyme supply over the years, additional reinforcement through plant enzymes may be advisable.

We propose in the "Ideal Diet," described on page 165, that the nutritional goal is for 30% of the vegetables and fruits that make up 75% of each day's food intake to be eaten raw. Supplementation with plant enzymes is appropriate even for those on this Ideal Diet. If the patient has not reached the Ideal Diet and eats greater quantities of cooked food, even more enzyme supplements should be taken.

THE CONNECTION BETWEEN ENZYME DEFICIENCY AND DISEASE

Enzymes are present in all living food. Plants progress through the natural growing and ripening process. Enzymes in plants govern this process which takes fruits and vegetables through the growing, maturing, ripening, and decomposition stages. Every living food has the enzymes necessary to begin, if not complete, the digestion of that food. When food is eaten, it should be digested from the inside out and from the outside in. When a piece of ripe fruit is eaten, the enzymes that control the ripening process within the fruit continue to function even after the fruit is taken into the body — from the inside out. At the same time, the body's digestive processes are acting on the fruit — digestion of the fruit takes place from the outside in. If the food that is consumed has no enzymes to assist in preparing the food for assimilation, the body itself is called upon to carry out the entire function which places additional, unnecessary stress on the entire system. Accumulated stress is referred to as aging, fatigue, exhaustion, or disease.

Disease is often attributed to external germs and bacteria invading the body, and much of science is dedicated to obliterating these substances. However, we must keep in mind that plants cannot grow without bacteria, fungi, or yeast. These properties can cause disease in man but they are vital to the overall picture of providing the materials (foods) man needs to survive.

Germs and bacteria are not the cause of disease. We are constantly exposed to and bombarded by microscopic organisms that cannot find a home in a healthy body. Disease occurs when timing, toxicity, or thoughts reduce the vitality of the body to allow invading scavengers to survive and flourish. Enzyme deficiencies contribute to both toxicity and inappropriate timing. If the enzymes of the food we eat have been destroyed, the digestive processes in the stomach cannot function as intended. Cooked food passes through the stomach and puts a tremendous drain on the internal enzyme systems of the pancreas. Without replenishment of enzymes that are available in raw fruits and vegetables, we not only put an increased demand on the internal enzyme system, we use up our internal enzymes at an alarming rate. Dr. Howell proposes that longevity and health are the result of a healthy enzyme system — when the enzyme supply is depleted, the body becomes "old," no matter what the age.[16] We can see that when the vitality of the body goes down as enzyme abuse continues, the body is subject to any of the many chronic degenerative diseases. As the body's vitality and resistance are lowered due to depletion of enzymes in the body, "scavengers" in the form of bacteria, viruses, fungi, or yeast find a home where they can be well-fed and can propagate in an environment of low vitality.

Disease is nothing more than the body's attempt to rid itself of morbific matter. The waste material that the body is no longer able to assimilate or eliminate in natural processes accumulates and provides hospitable surroundings for bacteria, viruses, and fungi to live and proliferate. Every bacteria was created to serve a perfect function for the benefit of man. However, this function is served by these scavengers when they are in the soil where they can assist in getting nitrogen into plants that man can eat raw. These same scavengers cause disease in man when they find a home in the organs of the body. If man's vitality is lowered to the same level as that of the soil, bacteria, viruses, and other predators have an open invitation to inhabit the body. Germs are not the cause of sickness — the body is sick before germs gain a foothold.

VITALITY OF FOOD

The enzymes in the food we eat represent the living quality. The vitality of the food we eat must always be higher than the vitality of the material we are trying to build, otherwise, we are trying to "build uphill" which is not possible for man. Plants can convert lesser vitality into greater. In the photosynthesis process, the amount of energy in glucose is greater than the amount of energy in each constituent part of carbon dioxide, water, light energy and chlorophyll. Man does not have the ability to generate more vitality than is replenished — man must eat food that has more vitality than he. The body will attain the same vitality as the vitality of the food we eat. If we continually eat lifeless, devitalized food, the vitality level of our body will eventually match that of the food. Yet we know that the body will do everything possible to maintain and sustain life. When the body is not furnished life-enriching enzymes through the food we eat, it will produce enzymes — without conscious thought — but there are limits to production capabilities.

Raw foods are the source of the vitality that allows the body to function at maximum efficiency and comfort. When the diet consists almost exclusively of cooked foods, little digestion takes place in the stomach and the pancreas must perform functions it was not originally designed to perform. We have stated that we attain the vitality level of the foods we eat. Consequently, when the diet is made up almost exclusively of cooked or processed substances, the pancreas is expected to perform the function of vital plant enzymes. The pancreas, however, is operating under the constraints of being nourished by low-vitality foods as well as being devoid of alkaline reserve minerals. Enzyme exhaustion and alkaline reserve depletion are co-conspirators in the progression of pain, reduced immunity, poor health, and chronic degenerative disease.

10

INDICATORS OF HEALTH

MONITORING HEALTH

We have been discussing how the intricate and synergistic relationships of the body's many systems affect metabolism, homeostasis, and overall health. We have seen that our dietary habits can lead to chronic degenerative disease if the alkaline reserves of the body are overtaxed. As a life-sustaining measure, the body will do what is necessary to neutralize excessive amounts of acid that are generated when high-protein foods are digested. The measures taken to offset this excess acid take care of the immediate problem. However, when these adaptive measures are the rule rather than the exception, they can lead to far-reaching long-term repercussions ranging from irritability and restlessness to osteoporosis, arthritis, cancer, AIDS, and other chronic degenerative diseases.

Recalling that the body's response is always appropriate to the stimuli, it is the doctor's role to help patients identify life style factors that contribute to the patient's physiological problems. Urinalysis can be used to reveal how the patient's body is responding to the food he eats and to determine the patient's current state of health.

Understanding the physiological processes that produce the various substances excreted in the urine can lead to accurate interpretation of urinalysis findings. Readily available reagent strips indicate the urine pH level as well as the presence of protein, glucose, ketones, bilirubin, blood, nitrates, and urobilinogen. This information, correlated with reports of variations in saliva pH readings during specific times of day, can provide the doctor with a comprehensive picture of the state of patients' overall health.

When the patient monitors and records the pH of both urine and saliva on a daily basis, he becomes an active participant on his journey to health rather than a passive passenger.

URINE pH

Urine pH indicates how a patient's body is responding to the food he ate the previous day and can help in the assessment of his total health. However, determining that the urine is alkaline has little diagnostic value until this piece of information is correlated with information indicating the reason for the alkalinity. If the urine is alkaline because ammonia and bicarbonate are present, very likely the patient will be experiencing bladder irritation or infection, muscle soreness, backache, joint stiffness, or allergy symptoms. Ammonia and bicarbonate in the urine can be the result of insufficient alkaline reserves. When the liver no longer has alkaline resources to neutralize acid, and sodium is not available to be combined with bicarbonate for reabsorption, ammonia and bicarbonate are eliminated in the urine.

If the urine is alkaline because the patient is a strict vegetarian, not only will the patient feel good but there will be no sign of bladder irritation or infection since the body has excess fixed alkaline reserves available to be eliminated.

It may be helpful to review what the body is trying to do when it excretes urine — it is getting rid of substances it can't use or that are detrimental. On a vegetable diet, natural waste products will be eliminated; on a high-meat diet, ammonia, bicarbonate, and perhaps protein will be excreted. Regardless of its condition, the body is doing the best it can, under the circumstances, to rid itself of waste from recent meals and snacks.

IMPLICATIONS OF URINE pH READINGS

A great deal of information can be gained about a patient by monitoring his urine as he follows a controlled dietary regimen. If the patient's urine pH initially shows an alkaline reaction, have him eat nothing but acid-ash forming food for two days. After the two days, he should collect the first specimen following at least five hours of sleep. A specimen registering pH 5.5 or less indicates an adequate alkaline reserve — that there is enough sodium to combine with sulfate and nitrate ions to form an acid salt. It also indicates that neither free bicarbonate ions nor ammonia is being excreted in the urine to give it an alkaline pH. This patient will readily respond to treatment since the body will heal itself on a priority basis and, in this instance, toxicity is not a priority and the energy needed for healing can be directed elsewhere.

If, however, the patient eats only acid-ash producing foods for two days and his urine shows a pH 8, a more serious situation exists. This tells you that his alkaline reserve is depleted and that bicarbonate and ammonia are in the urine giving it an alkaline reading — sodium is lacking, and acid salt cannot be formed. Protein may even be found in the urine because all of the buffer systems are overtaxed and unable to process the protein adequately. Protein in the urine is never Normal, but in this case it is absolutely Necessary. (See chart "Implications of Urine pH Readings" on page 185.)

Ammonia in the Urine

Although ammonia is produced by cells through metabolism, under normal conditions this ammonia is carried to the liver and converted to neutral urea. So the ammonia of deamination at the cellular level is not generally eliminated by the kidneys.

The kidney cells have the ability, in the presence of excess protein, to create and excrete ammonia directly into the urine. It is ammonia that is produced as a result of excess protein — not the ammonia produced by the other cells of the body — that makes the urine alkaline. Under normal levels of protein consumption, almost all cells of the body can convert ammonia into neutral urea for excretion in the urine.

Deamination is the removal of amino groups from protein and may occur in the kidneys when protein consumption persists. The ammonia that results from deamination will have a pH of 9.23, which is the pK of a 1% physiological solution of ammonia. When extracellular fluid contains a disproportionately high amount of ammonia, calcium and potassium reverse positions in relation to the cell membrane. The calcium may go into the cell (increasing the need to extract biological calcium from bones) and the potassium may come out of the cell into the blood, increasing the blood potassium level even though the patient is in a state of acidosis. When the extracellular fluid has a 7.4 pH, calcium is on the cell membrane; potassium is on the inside and the calcium on the outside. But the addition of more ammonia disturbs the delicate balance of this system. It is this ammonia solution that is responsible for a pH 8.0 or higher urine of the patient who eats only acid forming foods and whose alkaline reserve is totally depleted. This condition illustrates that apparent alkalosis is in reality a severe degree of acidosis.

Patient on Alkalizing Diet - Acid Urine

If a patient is on a diet of only alkalizing foods for two days — fruits and vegetables — and a check of the urine finds a pH of 5.5 or below, a rather complex picture is presented. First, you know that he has no alkaline reserve, but he does have enough acid in the stomach to metabolize the food into a form that can go directly to the cells where it is desperately needed. His body has not yet replenished the exhausted alkaline reserve but is sustaining itself in the current situation. If the patient continues to consume fruits and vegetables exclusively, the cellular demands for organic minerals will eventually be satisfied and the alkaline reserve will begin to be rebuilt and the urine pH will gradually increase from 5.5 to 6.8. The bank overdraft is satisfied and the account is being replenished, but the process may take from one to six months.

Patient on Alkalizing Diet - Alkaline Urine

If the patient eats fruits and vegetables for two days and the urine is pH 7.0, this means either that the alkaline reserve is adequate or that the cells cannot utilize the organic minerals. It may be that the minerals are metabolized well enough to get into the blood, but there is not yet an environment suitable for them to get inside the cells. This patient may need a supplement such as betaine hydrochloride or pancreatic enzymes to improve digestion and metabolism to the point at which the cells can accept the needed minerals. There may also be a problem of timing — the cells may simply need more time to regain the vitality necessary to accept the minerals. It may be six months before this patient will experience symptomatic change and begin to feel better.

A paradoxical situation arises from excess acidity in that the more acid the system of the individual the more acid supplementation such as betaine hydrochloride will be required to relieve symptoms. The reason for this is that the parietal cells (the acid producing cells) of a patient in this condition are so toxic that they cannot produce hydrochloric acid, which is the medium necessary to acidify the chyme before it enters the duodenum to encounter the alkaline bile and pancreatic enzymes.

Various organs and systems have different pH levels that span a range from pH 2 for the stomach contents to pH 8 for the bile and pancreatic enzymes. When these two divergent pH levels meet in the duodenum, a tremendous burst of energy is released. However, as the patient's health deteriorates, the differences among the acidity of the saliva, digestive, stomach, and duodenum fluids are reduced and the energy is not released.

MODIFYING pH THROUGH DIET

If a patient shows an alkaline urine pH due to bicarbonate and ammonia, particular care must be taken in changing this person's diet. Fruit intake should be kept low and vegetables should be added to his current diet without specifically restricting the foods he is accustomed to eating. Fruits and vegetables provide a fixed base which ordinarily would be very soothing to the bladder. But when these alkalizing foods are introduced and the urine is already alkaline from bicarbonate and ammonia produced by the body in processing excess protein, the abnormality of the urine is exaggerated and the patient will likely experience a rather severe bladder irritation.

The ammonia that is present in these situations can be particularly irritating to the urinary tract. A patient whose urine is highly alkaline due to the presence of ammonia, bicarbonate, and protein must drink one to four glasses of cranberry juice daily to neutralize the alkaline urine. At the same time, the patient must begin to eat cooked vegetables and continue to do so as the body slowly rebuilds its depleted alkaline reserve. This is an example of the situation where the patient's system must be acidified while it is being alkalized.

In evaluating the patient's health on a crisis basis, bilirubin in the urine is the most reliable indicator of the degree of physical distress; in evaluating the patient's health on a non-crisis basis, pH is the best indicator. For the patient who expresses highly acid pH levels, the objective is to manage the treatment in such a manner as to move the urine and saliva pH to natural levels without the patient feeling worse in the process.

SALIVA pH

The purpose of urinalysis is to gain information about the patient which will assist in determining the treatment that will help him to become more healthy. However, urinalysis will not tell the entire story any more than will any other single test, although it does reveal more than most. Checking the pH of saliva in addition to the pH of urine yields some very significant information that enhances the value of the urinalysis.

The first urine specimen of the morning is the most revealing in terms of how well the body handled the food that was eaten the day before. Urine pH readings can change each morning depending upon the patient's condition and the food he ate the day before. Saliva pH, however, is a better indicator of the patient's overall health; it reveals the current condition of the alkaline reserve, and we have seen throughout this study that the state of the alkaline reserve is directly connected with the patient's diet of past months and years.

Recall that the liver is the alkaline reserve storehouse; saliva pH can be the best indicator of intracellular liver pH and of the availability of alkaline reserve minerals. Saliva pH also gives the most reliable information on the pH of the intracellular and extracellular fluids.

Saliva pH readings taken each morning upon awakening will remain relatively constant from day to day. However, saliva pH can be altered instantly during the day after eating. In a healthy person, saliva pH changes in an upward direction toward alkalinity, never downward, before returning to its normal reading. Saliva pH should never be lower than 6.8 which is the pK of the phosphate buffer system. This pH should rise immediately after the patient has eaten, or, literally, if he even thinks about eating.

As an experiment, test your own saliva pH. Then think, graphically, of cutting into a firm, lemon that is dripping with tart, sour, mouth-puckering juice. See yourself squeezing some of that juice into a spoon, putting the pulpy golden liquid into your mouth, and feel your salivary glands respond sharply as the tangy juice envelopes your tongue and teeth.

Now, test your saliva pH again.

If you are relatively healthy and have a reasonably vivid imagination, you will probably find the second reading to be approximately 8 on the pH scale. This indicates the speed at which the saliva pH can react. It also serves to illustrate how dramatically thoughts can affect saliva pH and, by the same token, affect total body function. If thoughts can instantly change saliva pH by two points, imagine how heart rate, blood pressure, and other physiological functions can respond to mental stimuli. In the experiment with the lemon, negative thoughts were not involved — distasteful perhaps, but not life-threatening. This parlor-game experiment with the lemon illustrates the power that thoughts (which are strictly internal stimulation) can have on physical reactions.

Since saliva pH is an indicator of intracellular pH, saliva readings should never be below the pK of the phosphate buffer system, 6.8. The most accurate reading of saliva pH is recorded immediately upon awakening — after sleeping at least five hours and before brushing the teeth. It is during sleep that the body removes waste and is in an anabolic state restoring and replenishing the body. If the patient has a saliva pH of 5.5 at this time and only 5.6 after eating, you know that this person has no alkaline reserve and that his body is devoid of the minerals necessary to process food properly — his body cannot adequately respond to the physiological crisis of handling food. (See chart "Implications of Saliva pH Readings" on page 187.)

The more acidic the food that is eaten, the more rapid the response of the alkaline reserve, and the higher the saliva pH should be following the meal. Since the saliva enzyme ptyalin works optimally at pH 8.5, acid is a threat to the normal alkaline pH of the mouth. When a healthy person with adequate alkaline reserves takes a bite of highly acid lemon, the saliva pH drops sharply for an instant but returns almost immediately to 8.5. The ideal saliva pH pattern is 6.8 upon awakening, 7.0 before eating, and 8.5 following breakfast. In order to assess the state of the patient's alkaline reserve, it is necessary to have both "Before Meal" and "After Meal" readings. The amount of change in pH is equally as important as the numbers themselves.

As a patient becomes more acid in general (physically and/or mentally) his saliva will also become more acid creating an environment conducive to harboring bacteria that cause tooth decay. If the alkaline reserve is lacking, saliva is acid and lemon juice would adversely effect tooth enamel because the body could not respond naturally to the influx of additional acid.

Saliva pH should rise at least one point immediately after drinking lemon water. The speed at which the saliva readings change and the amount of change give an idea of the condition of the patient's alkaline reserve. Even if no change in the pH is recorded, or if it decreases, valuable information is gained. Since saliva pH is an indicator of intracellular pH, the first saliva pH readings of the morning will vary only minutely from day to day. It will take weeks or months of a more healthful diet before changes in the awakening reading can be effected.

Dietary changes should be approached with utmost caution. If the patient is asymptomatic but his saliva and urine pH are both low, the doctor is in a precarious situation. Any corrections in the diet will begin to alter the pH to a more favorable condition but will almost certainly make the person feel worse. It is important that the patient understands this before any dietary changes are attempted. Unpleasant initial reactions cause many diet corrections to fail. If a person begins a new diet and feels worse after a few days, he will give up the whole idea, go back to his normal eating habits and feel better, but the problem will remain unresolved.

The reason the patient feels worse after eliminating stimulating substances such as coffee, sugar, or protein from his diet is that there is a time lag before the body is again governed by its own internal hormonal control. The body is accustomed to stimulation and it takes time for it to function comfortably without it. Even the best programs of dietary change will often produce temporary unpleasant responses. The patient should fully understand why this is occurring and be prepared for it at the outset.

EMOTIONS AND SALIVA pH

Saliva pH readings also indicate the status of extracellular pH, and we know that the pK of extracellular fluid is 6.1. Saliva pH lower than 6.1 indicates that the body cannot maintain the required minimum pH while handling stress.

Variations of the first morning saliva pH readings that range between 6.6 and 7.2 over a period of time are of little significance. However, if the patient's saliva pH is 6.0 upon awakening and it goes to 7.2 after a meal and stays there, you can assume that this is a physical response to an emotional situation. Mental or emotional stress of the patient stimulates the body in the same manner as the ingestion of food. The difference is that when the food is processed the emergency is over; but an emotional situation is ongoing and the body is forced to maintain a constant state of readiness to meet the emergency. In this situation, a person may sleep poorly and have a high saliva pH in the morning. However, if the saliva pH remains the same after a meal as it was prior to eating, you know that the pH before eating was a false emergency reading. The pH may be 5.8 before a meal and 6.0 after if the individual has been under emotional stress for a long period of time; or it can be 7.2 before eating and 7.6 following, indicating an acute emotional stress situation.

If saliva pH readings vary greatly on arising each morning, it is almost certain that anxiety is influencing the individual's physiology. For example, if the patient's before-breakfast morning saliva pH readings for a week are

Monday	5.5
Tuesday	6.2
Wednesday	6.8
Thursday	5.8
Friday	5.5
Saturday	7.2

you could conclude that this patient is extremely acid with a saliva pH of 5.5, but continued stress gives a reading of 7.2 indicating that even during sleep, emergency physiology exists. Bodily functions respond dramatically to thoughts as illustrated by the lemon demonstration.

11

CORRELATED FINDINGS

ADDITIONAL INDICATORS

We have, to this point, been focusing primarily on urinalysis indicators that are closely connected to the effects of excess protein consumption on the body. We should keep in mind, however, that there are additional indicators available to us to correlate with urinalysis findings. In this chapter we will look at some of these indicators and the roles they play in evaluating our patients' health.

GLUCOSE

Sugar in the urine, or glucosuria, is the result of a very complex biochemical process that may have little relationship to sugar intake. Sugar in the urine indicates a problem related to glucose metabolism that is probably associated with insulin. However, it does not necessarily mean that insulin production is deficient. In fact, recent studies have shown that diabetic patients produce normal to high amounts of insulin.[1]

It is helpful to view sugar in the urine as a brilliant reaction by the body to a potentially fatal situation. It may be difficult to think of a pathological condition such as sugar in the urine as being a life-saving function; however, if the patient is diabetic, as long as his kidneys are still able to filter enough sugar out of the blood, the blood sugar level will not rise to a point that would result in diabetic coma and possibly death. Sugar in the urine is certainly not Natural and is never Normal, but, in these cases, it is absolutely Necessary — the patient's total health picture must be considered in evaluating or interpreting any test results, including sugar in the urine.

Generally, the medical approach to treating a patient whose urinalysis reveals sugar being eliminated is to raise the level of insulin in the blood by injections. Although this may alleviate symptoms, it does not solve the problem. Symptoms of diabetes result when cells are unable to function properly.

Insulin

The primary role of insulin is to transport glucose through the cell wall. This function is accomplished most effectively in an extracellular fluid environment of pH 7.8 to 8.0.[2] If the fluid becomes too acid, a normal amount of insulin cannot be effective, but glucose can be forced through the cell wall by additional insulin administered by injection. However, insulin that is produced normally will be adequate and function effectively if the acid level of the extracellular fluid is reduced.

When a person eats a meal, his blood sugar level rises. Within about an hour, two-thirds of the available sugar is stored in the liver and the remaining one-third is stored in muscle cells. If the blood sugar level falls, the glucose stored in the liver is available for use; however, the glucose that is stored in the muscle cells cannot be liberated to increase blood sugar — it must be used by the muscles.

Hypoglycemia

In evaluating a patient with hypoglycemia, it is helpful to observe the timing of the hypoglycemic reaction to determine whether an insulin condition or another hormonal imbalance is involved. A reaction of fatigue, sleepiness, dizziness, or loss of the ability to concentrate that occurs immediately after eating is an indication of the presence of too much insulin as a result of too much white sugar or other highly refined carbohydrates. This overproduction stimulates an immediate intense physiological response that is followed quickly by an equally intense period of physical exhaustion. A reaction that occurs two hours after eating indicates that the liver is unable to get the stored glucose back into the blood; this is a hormonal situation possibly involving the pituitary and adrenal glands. As a generalization, we can say that if the hypoglycemic reaction occurs within two hours after eating, it is an insulin problem; if it occurs more than two hours after eating, it is another hormonal problem that does not involve insulin and may indicate that either the message system to the liver is faulty or the liver is unable to respond properly because of cellular congestion.

A word of caution: Hypoglycemia diagnosis requires a six-hour glucose tolerance test that is correlated with clinical findings and patient history. **Hypoglycemia cannot be diagnosed by urinalysis.**

KETONES

Ketones are acetone bodies that are present in normal urine in very small amounts.

Ketones are formed when carbohydrate intake is reduced (such as during a fast or rigid diet) and the body is forced to metabolize some of its stored fat. Ketones are then carried by the blood to extrahepatic tissue where further degradation occurs. Ketonuria results when either the liver produces an excessive amount of ketones or the extrahepatic tissue is unable to process and degrade them. Ketonuria may be expected to occur in acidosis of diabetes mellitis, starvation, normal and toxic pregnancies, after ether anesthesia, and often in alkalosis that is an advanced state of acidosis.

The fat that is metabolized to form ketones is the product of food that has already been digested and individualized and is, in effect, perfect food. With food intake restricted, less energy is needed for digestion and assimilation leaving more energy for healing. The best healing environment for the body is when it is in a slight state of ketosis.

In the treatment of yeast infections, arthritis, or any of the chronic degenerative diseases, detoxification occurs most rapidly when the patient's urine shows a trace of ketones. The level must be kept at a trace and monitored carefully, especially when the patient is attempting to lose weight or to break a habit. Keeping the patient in a very slight degree of ketosis can generally be accomplished by allowing him nothing more than one or two bananas a day. It is best (especially for a diabetic) to keep the urine pH above 5.8 - 6.0 while there is a trace of ketones in the urine.

BLOOD

A brief review of kidney function will be helpful in understanding the occurrence of blood in the urine.

The glomeruli of the kidneys are clusters of capillaries within a thin wall. These glomeruli have the ability to take substances from the blood in the vessels and, at some point further along the line within the kidney, to reclaim substances such as sodium, bicarbonate, and other vital properties. The substances taken back into the vessels are recirculated.

The kidneys perform three basic functions:

First, they **remove substances such as urobilinogen from the blood**. However, since urobilinogen is an abnormal constituent of blood there is no mechanism to reclaim it and it passes into the urine.

Second, the kidneys **maintain thresholds**. If the amount of any of the many substances normally found in the blood becomes excessive, the glomeruli will reclaim only as much as is needed to meet the body's current demands and requirements. The excess is eliminated in the urine.

The third function of the kidneys is **filtration**, which is illustrated by its relationship to red blood cells. These cells are so large, vital, and of such composition that, in healthy people, they never get into the glomeruli filtrate but remain in the vascular system. Consequently, red blood cells should not be found in the urine. Occasionally, blood will be caught accidentally in the specimen of a female during menstruation, but this is not a pathological indicator. When this occurs, the urine should be checked at another time of the cycle.

Blood in the urine may signal severe infection, injury, or trauma to the kidney or bladder and should be thoroughly investigated by additional tests and procedures to establish an exact cause. Urine that contains blood should be re-checked daily during treatment until blood is no longer present.

Hemolyzed red blood cells, if found in large numbers, could indicate a greater than average breakdown of red blood cells, or perhaps a hemolytic transfusion. The most common cause of hemolyzed cells in the urine is that the specimen is not fresh and the blood it contains has already undergone lysis.

CHOLESTEROL

The role cholesterol plays in nutrition has been widely disputed and discussed by both professionals and laymen in recent years. One of the greatest sources of confusion comes from the similarity between the cholesterol found in eggs and other foods and the cholesterol that is in the blood stream — they are not the same. In fact, in one case with which I am familiar, a patient was put on a diet of only eggs, and his serum cholesterol level decreased.

Cholesterol is a fat-like substance found in eggs, brain tissue, milk, animal fats, and oils. Cholesterol is also manufactured by the body. Although there is diversity of opinion concerning the value or danger of cholesterol, it should not be considered to be a foreign substance. On the contrary, it should be seen as a normal physiological substance necessary for manufacturing some vitamins and hormones as well as for metabolizing fats. It is only when we force the body to digest highly refined, high-calorie foods that cholesterol is manufactured in amounts that become a problem. We need cholesterol to live!

High serum cholesterol develops as a result of eating too many refined foods — processed, synthetic foods — highly refined "dead" foods that cause the body to produce excess cholesterol and to form fat. In order to reduce blood serum cholesterol, the intake of processed and refined foods — bread, cakes, spaghetti, instant mashed potatoes, and cereals for example — should be reduced or eliminated and, at the same time, the amount of fruits and vegetables should be increased.

ASCORBIC ACID

Ascorbic acid levels in the urine will increase if the patient is taking heavy doses of vitamin C or is eating large quantities of fruit. Excess vitamin C eliminated in the urine poses no threat to the patient.

Readings of 0 to 10 milligrams per deciliter of ascorbic acid in the urine are considered normal.

NITRITES

Nitrites in the urine can indicate a bladder infection. Nitrites are salts of nitric acid produced by bacterial action on nitrates that have been consumed in bacon or other processed food. It is not unusual to find nitrates in the urine when these foods are eaten. However, nitrites in the urine indicate that reducing bacteria are present in the bladder and the patient should be instructed to drink one to four glasses of cranberry juice per day. The patient should continue to drink cranberry juice, even if he isn't experiencing pain, as long as nitrites appear in the urine, and the urine should be monitored until the nitrites are no longer present.

SPECIFIC GRAVITY

The specific gravity of water, 1.000, is used as the standard against which the specific gravity of other liquids is measured. In urinalysis, specific gravity is a measure of the thickness of urine.

Normal specific gravity of urine is considered to be 1.008 to 1.025, just slightly thicker than water.[3] Very low urine specific gravity readings could indicate one of two things: the person has just consumed a large quantity of water, coffee, tea, or watermelon; or, the kidneys are unable to filter properly and are passing only water with no solids. If the latter is the cause, a severe kidney condition is indicated and imminent kidney failure is possible.

A urine specific gravity reading of 1.030 indicates either the presence of protein or sugar, or that the kidneys have been concentrating the urine more than necessary. In either case, the urine is too thick — a condition which puts additional stress on this vital organ.

A high specific gravity reading indicates toxicity or inadequate fluid intake. The body will retain fluids in order to dilute toxic materials, protein, or glucose and to maintain normal intracellular osmolarity. Fluid retention (edema) that is exhibited symmetrically — such as when both legs or both ankles are swollen — can be attributed to toxicity of the body. Asymmetrical swelling — one leg, one ankle, or one hand — is generally caused by neurological interference or an obstruction in the circulatory system.

A urine sample with a specific gravity of 1.025 will probably show a trace of protein. This reading is being seen more and more in our society, and since "normal" appears to be determined by the frequency with which a given condition is manifest in asymptomatic people; both a trace of protein and an increase in specific gravity measurement may be considered to be normal in the near future. Neither of these conditions is natural.

If glucose is the cause of a high specific gravity reading, ketones will generally be found. However, if neither protein nor sugar is present to account for the high reading, the patient should be instructed to drink large amounts of distilled or reverse osmotic water to dilute the urine and relieve stress on the kidneys.

12

THE IMPORTANCE OF CORRECT EATING AND EXERCISE

CALORIES AND FOODS

In our weight-conscious society, food and calories are almost synonymous to many Americans although, actually, the number of calories consumed may not be as important in a weight control program as is the type of food eaten.

"Calorie" can be defined as the amount of heat required to raise the temperature of one gram of water one degree centigrade. The calories referred to when talking about human nutrition are kilocalories, or large calories. A large calorie is the amount of heat needed to raise the temperature of 1000 grams of water 1° Centigrade[1] and is the unit we will be concerned with here. Essentially, a calorie is the unit used in referring to the amount of energy used in metabolizing a certain amount of food.

The number of calories in a portion of food has almost nothing to do with that food being "fattening." You can actually lose weight by eating high-calorie foods. I had a patient who lost three pounds in one week eating only almonds, avocadoes and figs — all high in calories. I do not recommend such a diet and cite it only to emphasize that the calorie content is not as critical to weight loss as the public has been led to believe. The most important factor is how the body uses the food, not how many calories are consumed. For example, baked potatoes and macaroni have approximately the same number of calories and both are classified as starches; however, there the similarity ends.[2] Although they both eventually supply glucose to the cells, the overall effect these two foods have on the body is vastly different. The body utilizes all of the potato in a stress-free manner, while physiological processing of macaroni, that has few enzymes, vitamins, or minerals, puts stress on several systems of the body. To explain this, it is important to understand how the body uses food.

THE FUNCTION OF FOOD

We eat food in order to (1) supply physical and mental energy, (2) repair and replace worn tissue, and (3) supply materials with which the body manufactures hormones, enzymes and other substances. Regardless of the ultimate purpose of the food, the body is designed to operate on whole, complete foods. For example, a baked potato is a whole food if the skin as well as the inside is eaten. The body can use it all because the outer part of the potato near the skin provides the vitamins and other substances which the body uses to make the enzymes needed to digest the inside of the potato. Peeled potatoes, such as mashed potatoes, are not whole, complete foods because some of the needed vitamins and enzyme precursors have been removed with the potato peelings.

The body's infinite intelligence decides that the mashed potato isn't good enough to use but is too good to discard, consequently, it is stored as fat. When the whole potato (complete with skin) is eaten, the body utilizes the ingredients it needs and eliminates the waste as nature intended. No fragments remain, therefore, no fat is stored.

The important thing to remember is that calorie intake should not be restricted in an effort to lose weight — the kind of food that is eaten is more significant. A diet that includes mostly fruits and vegetables (as recommended in this book) will provide the kinds of food that will not only help patients to reach and maintain weight appropriate to each individual but will also provide the foods the body needs and can use most effectively.

PROTEIN IN FOODS

Many patients claim that they don't feel satisfied unless they eat meat with their meal. For those who are accustomed to it, meat has a high satiety value — it satisfies the appetite. It also keeps the body busy for about five hours during the processing of the meal even though the meal may not have provided all of the nutrients the body needed. The meat acts as an external stimulant in that the stimulation comes from the increased metabolic activity necessary to process the meat for assimilation and elimination.

As the diet is changed to more fruits and vegetables, hunger for meat will diminish and ultimately disappear. We have said that after a period of time, those who have given up meat find that meat has given them up — they lose their desire for meat as their bodies begin to operate from internal control which is governed by the hormonal system. When this natural control is reinstituted, the liver and adrenal glands will raise the blood sugar level at the appropriate time without being bolstered by a "food fix" between meals.

A popular misconception is that protein comes only from meat, eggs, and dairy products such as cheese. In reality, it is almost impossible to eat anything in the vegetable kingdom that does not contain some protein. Any whole, natural vegetable or fruit contains protein — usually about 1.5%. Although the concentration is low, this protein is completely usable and does not stress the body in any way during the digestion and assimilation processes. There is one important qualification, however: the vegetables and fruits must be whole and natural. Any food that has been altered or processed does not qualify as either "whole" or "natural." Not only can altered or processed foods stress the body during the process of digestion, they may be incomplete and lacking in the nutrients the body needs.

FOOD COMBINING

Even an excellent selection of foods can be rendered unsatisfactory if the foods of a meal are combined improperly. A complete discussion of the benefits of properly combining foods for various meals is beyond the scope of this book, however, the Food Combining Chart shown on page 173 and a few rules may prove helpful.

The food combining chart illustrates those foods or food groups that are compatible with each other and those that should not be eaten at the same meal. You will note that some food groups are bordered by two lines, others by only one line. In selecting foods for a meal, combine only those that are in food groups separated by only one line. If in "moving" from one food group to another, you "pass through" another food group, this may count as "two lines" even though the lines are not together. For instance, foods in the "Protein" group can be combined with both those in the "Vegetable-Salad" group and the "Acid Fruit" and "Semi-Acid" groups — only one line is crossed from one group to the other. However, when those in the "Protein" group are combined with those in the "Dairy" group, two lines were crossed. "Sweet Fruit" and "Melons" are bordered by two lines and should always be eaten alone.

The numerical evaluations assigned indicate the alkalizing or acidifying effect the particular food has on the body. Foods showing positive numbers have an alkalizing effect; foods showing negative numbers have an acidifying effect. The higher the number, the more intense the reaction; that is, molasses at +2507.1 is considerably more alkalizing than white potatoes at + 26.3. And, on the other end of the spectrum, sausage at -160.7 is more acidifying than pork chops at -9.9. The following guidelines are generalizations of the more detailed chart.

- Protein and starches require completely different digestive environments and should never be eaten together.

- Protein should never be eaten with fruit.

- Starches and fruits should not be eaten together.

- Begin each meal with something raw to allow the body to start manufacturing enzymes that can be carried over and used to produce personalized enzymes.

- Melons should be eaten alone — never in combination with other food.

- Milk is not recommended. For those who choose to drink milk, it should be raw and consumed by itself — never in combination with other foods.

- Liquids, including water, should not be consumed with meals as these dilute the digestive fluids. If the patient is thirsty, it is because he is eating improper foods.

WATER

Part of our cultural heritage glorifies pure, untreated water — the kind you get from Uncle Homer's well. However, I question whether this "pure" water is really good for us. Well water contains minerals — inorganic minerals that, as we have seen, are held together by ionic bonds that the body is not able to break apart. I believe that the body does not use any inorganic substances from water; minerals that are neither needed nor used must be stored in the body until they can be eliminated. "Hard" water contains dissolved minerals that the body must filter out — another energy consuming process. In "soft" water, the calcium and iron salts have been replaced with sodium of sodium chloride, and the excess inorganic sodium interferes with natural organic sodium in the body. This explains why soft water, whether naturally or artificially softened, can be more harmful to the body than hard water.

The best kind of water for the body is the water contained in fruits and vegetables. When a patient changes his diet to include predominantly fruits and vegetables, he is often surprised at how little additional water he needs to keep his body satisfied.

Pure rain water would be the second best source of water. However, since "pure" rainwater is no longer available anywhere in our polluted world, distilled or reverse osmosis water are suitable substitutes.

DISTILLED WATER

Distilled water contains no minerals; it is, in essence, a substance that is not encountered in nature and is foreign to the body. Some patients resist drinking distilled water because they believe that it leaches minerals from the body. This is an accurate assessment but the leaching is an advantage rather than a disadvantage. The advantage is that distilled water can absorb and remove hard, ionic minerals from the body rather than add to the unwanted store.

In a rather complex chemical process, minerals are carried between the hydrogen and oxygen atoms in non-distilled water. Distilled water, on the other hand, is "empty" in that these spaces are not filled; however, given the opportunity, they will be. When distilled water is taken into the body, some of the unusable, inorganic minerals that have been stored in the body will fill the available spaces in the distilled water and will be eliminated.

Inorganic minerals that are leached from the body by the distilled water serve no useful physiological purpose. In fact, they interfere with normal physiological function. Drinking distilled water will help to rid the body of some of these accumulated "hard" minerals. Organic, covalent minerals are attached to an acid (as in fruit) or to a protein, and as such are not leached from the body by the distilled water.

When the leaching process has gone on for a period of time, a spoonful of fresh lemon juice should be added to each glass of distilled water the patient drinks. The lemon juice will not only make the water taste better, it will afford the body the chance to replace inorganic minerals with organic minerals that help to avert fatigue that could result from sudden mineral loss. The lemon juice should be fresh; reconstituted lemon juice is not an adequate substitute.

REVERSE OSMOSIS WATER

Reverse osmosis (RO) water is preferable to distilled water for drinking since it has not been boiled and has more life in it. The RO process is a development of space-age technology that filters water through a screen or membrane so fine that only the molecules of water can pass. Most minerals and impurities are filtered out, and chlorine, a gas that can permeate the membrane, can be removed by adding a charcoal filter to the RO unit.

CHLORINATED WATER

The least desirable water for human consumption is the water provided by most cities and other municipal districts. "City" water contains chlorine, a powerful oxidizing agent, that is not beneficial to the body and may be harmful.

Water or other liquid should not be consumed with meals. Liquids interfere with enzymatic function by diluting the medium in which digestive enzymes operate. When fruits and vegetables constitute most of the diet, thirst is minimal. A patient who is thirsty following a meal has eaten the wrong foods.

EXERCISE

Health conscious patients frequently see exercise and nutrition as basic elements leading to good health and longevity. While this may be true, strenuous exercise can cause unexpected physical problems if the patient's body is in or near a state of acidosis. Understanding the relationship between exercise and the body's pH is particularly important to both professional and amateur athletes.

Recall that the body is an alkaline organism by design and an acid organism by function. Muscles generate acid during exercise — lactic acid — which the heart can use as fuel. However, if the patient's acid level is already high due to a continuous high-protein diet, the lactic acid produced adds to stress on the body and heart.

No one who is a moderate to heavy meat eater should engage in strenuous exercise if his urine pH is either very high or very low. Extreme pH readings usually indicate that the body is very acid and that the alkaline reserve is being depleted. The production of additional acid from any source — diet or exercise — results in excess hydrogen ions that could stress the body beyond its ability to cope. Those who are on high protein diets and whose urine pH registers above 7 risk serious problems if they engage in strenuous physical exercise such as jogging. Until the patient can maintain an acid pH urine after an acid ash meal, he should not jog. When the urine pH level is brought down to 5 or below, this patient can safely jog moderately. However, those over 40 years of age should be especially careful to maintain saliva pH at 6.2 to assure that they have sufficient alkaline reserve available to handle strenuous exercise.

It is not uncommon to read a news report of a professional athlete or well-conditioned amateur athlete dying of a heart attack while exercising. The physical fitness world was shocked by the sudden death of Jim Fixx, author and authority on jogging. Fixx, from all outward appearances in excellent physical condition and definitely not overweight, died while jogging. In his best-selling *Jim Fixx's Second Book of Running*, Fixx pointed out that he had altered his diet gradually, was eating less meat than he had previously and neither missed it nor noticed any adverse physical effects.[3] Considering his level of physical activity, it could be conjectured that his life may have been extended had he reduced his acid-ash producing food intake more substantially and sooner. Jogging-track deaths can often been seen as the impact of vigorous physical exercise on a body already in an advanced state of acidosis.

Perhaps more common to our culture is the overweight patient who eats a big meal of acid-ash producing food topped off with a cup of coffee and a cigarette — a routine that substantially increases the acidity of his body. If the meal is followed by a period of strenuous exertion, the patient becomes a prime candidate for a heart attack.

WALKING AND CONTRALATERAL MOVEMENT

Walking is the exercise preferred for all who are able, and especially for those on high protein diets. Walking should be at a pace that does not raise the heart rate above 120 beats per minute. This type of activity will exercise the muscles but will not tax the cardiovascular system. The objective is to exercise in a way that will not generate additional acid in quantities that would subject the body to an environment it cannot handle. As the diet and general health improve, the amount and intensity of exercise can be increased.

We recommend that all patients walk for exercise and that they understand the importance and principle of contralateral movement. As the name implies, contralateral movement involves coordination of opposite sides of the body, i.e., the right arm and left leg, and the left arm and right leg. This movement is accomplished in walking when the left arm swings forward as a step is taken with the right leg and the right arm swings forward as a step is taken with the left leg. Walking with contralateral movement is not only excellent exercise but, more important, it is the one action that reorganizes and re-times the body. It is nature's way of returning bodily functions to normal.

Contralateral movement is critical to the total health of a patient. Swimming can be contralateral when backstroke or freestyle strokes are used and, in freestyle, the head is turned both ways for breathing. All exercises, including other swimming strokes, weight lifting or health club activities, should be followed by a brief, brisk walk to give the body a chance to normalize.

An illustration of the inherent sensitivity of the body to contralateral movement involved one of my staff members. She had purchased a sophisticated exercise bicycle that allowed for movement of both arms and legs. She mentioned that each time she used the equipment she developed a headache. Since this response is contrary to the effect contralateral movement should have, we investigated. Careful analysis of muscle action revealed that pulling on the handle bars did not provide contralateral exercise, but pushing the handle bars resulted in true contralateral movement. The staff member altered her method of exercise and the headache problem was eliminated.

Contralateral walking exercise is suitable for patients of all ages. However, carrying objects that restrict arm mobility while walking will not be as beneficial since this impairs contralateral movement. Also, wearing a radio or tape player with a headset while jogging or walking, as is currently in general vogue, is not recommended as this interferes with re-timing the muscles of the body. The important point to remember is that walking should be done in the manner that will give the greatest benefit to the body.

ACUTE PAIN

The source of acute pain is not always obvious. It can stem from an injury, disease, abuse (either intentional or unintentional) of the body, or from emotional distress. A thorough record of the patient's history can help to determine the cause of pain.

We have seen that pH and body chemistry are interrelated and may be associated with acute pain. If the patient's pain level increases during the day, the timing of synergistic or antagonistic muscles may be involved. The muscles may be working against themselves or perhaps, in a situation known as "recruiting," they are called upon to do a job they were not designed to do. Muscles used in this way will eventually register pain.

Toxicity can also be involved in acute pain. Patients who awaken in the morning in a great deal of pain but the pain subsides as the day goes on may be experiencing the results of toxicity. As the circulatory and excretory functions of the body improve with activity, this patient will feel better.

Excess alkalinity also causes unpleasant symptoms — colds, virus infections, bladder infections, and shingles are all manifestations of excess alkalinity, not excess acidity. However, the alkalinity is due to ammonia and bicarbonate rather than to organic minerals. As stated throughout this book, if a person continues to eat a diet high in meat, his system will first become acid, then alkaline. When the excess alkalinity reaches a level intolerable to the body, the patient will experience either a cold, bladder infection, or some other acute cleansing procedure. The orange juice usually consumed in these situations actually makes the condition worse since it increases the body's cleansing action.

The patient in this situation or in acute pain needs to let his body run itself. Drinking several glasses of cranberry juice a day will make the patient feel better by neutralizing the excess bicarbonate and ammonia and alleviating some of the symptoms of a bladder infection. A problem arises if the patient assumes that he developed the infection because he wasn't drinking enough cranberry juice and he drinks it every day to ward off further infections. Cranberry juice is one of the few fruit substances that has an acidifying effect on the body, consequently, this juice adds to the body's already over-acid condition.

Cells congested with bicarbonate and ammonia (indicated by an alkaline urine pH) cannot function properly; however, adding alkalizing minerals at this point will not be effective. The body must first be acidified before it can begin to alkalize. Two or three days of nothing but cranberry juice is usually sufficient to lessen pain. Following that, the patient should add generous quantities of green beans to his diet to begin the process of alkalizing his body.

A patient may experience severe leg cramps after changing from a high-protein diet to a more healthful regimen. Although this may appear to be contradictory, an understanding of the physiology involved will clarify this statement. A patient who has been on a high-protein, low-vegetable diet for an extended period of time will have depleted his alkaline reserve. As a result, the body is taking calcium from the bones to use as an acid neutralizer. When the body is no longer required to process large quantities of protein, the calcium extracting stimulus is removed but the patient is deficient in calcium. This results in leg cramps that will continue until the body has sufficient minerals from vegetables and fruits to replenish the depleted reserves. Unfortunately, the calcium will not be immediately available to prevent muscle cramps after fruits and vegetables replace protein in the diet. Long-standing conditions can take time to correct.

13

DIETS TO IMPROVE HEALTH

CORRECTING DIETS

We have cautioned against changing patients' diets so rapidly that they develop uncomfortable symptoms such as a cold, flu, or burning on urination. Each of the three diets described here — Modified, Transitional, and Ideal — is designed to help patients, according to each individual's level of health, to improve that level under controlled conditions. The Modified Diet should be followed by patients who are changing from a high-protein or junk food diet to one that includes more fruits and vegetables. The Transitional Diet is for patients whose bodies have become acclimated to processing more healthful foods and whose health is gradually improving. The Ideal Diet is a maintenance diet for patients who have achieved normal, natural physiological function and who intend to sustain their level of improved health.

MODIFIED DIET

Patients who have followed either the SAD or junk food diets for long periods of time should not make immediate drastic alterations to their eating habits. Those who suddenly embrace "nutrition religion" often find that unpleasant symptoms that accompany an abrupt change to be justification for returning to their former eating patterns. By having the patient "modify" his diet by adding vegetables and fruits, the body can adapt more smoothly to the more healthful foods. The patient is not asked to "give up" anything he is currently eating and enjoys; people ordinarily include in their eating habits only those foods they like. When the patient is instructed merely to add other foods to those they are already eating, he may not even view the addition as a part of being "put on a diet."

The Modified Diet is to initiate dietary changes for the very ill patient whose body is highly toxic. Again, this patient's diet should not be changed radically or suddenly. He should follow his usual eating pattern EXCEPT that he should ADD one serving of vegetables and one piece of fruit per day. He will also need an essence of barley extract, a plant enzyme, and egg calcium supplements. If he is experiencing bladder irritation or infection, cranberry juice should be added to his diet only while the irritation or infection is present. The patient should continue on this diet (without cranberry juice if he is symptom free) until his pH readings indicate improvement or stabilization.

Modify Existing Diet by Adding:	One serving of vegetables per day One piece of fruit per day
Supplementation:	Essence of barley extract, Betaine hydrochloride with pancreatic enzymes, and plant enzymes, Egg Calcium
	Cranberry juice, only if bladder irritation or infection is present

TRANSITIONAL DIET

The Transitional Diet serves as a bridge — or transition — between the modification of a long-standing diet and the diet that is ideal for maintaining the highest level of health. This diet is instituted when saliva and urine pH readings indicate that the patient's body is beginning to respond; that is, when the pH readings indicate his alkaline reserve is beginning to be replenished. The patient is still not asked to "give up" anything. He can continue with his regular diet but he can increase vegetable and fruit consumption even more. One meal a day should be only vegetables, and a second serving of fruit can be added. Supplementation may be reduced.

As the patient remains on the Transitional Diet, saliva and urine pH readings will improve. The improved pH readings are a reflection of the normal working of the body. Fruit and vegetable consumption can be increased and supplementation may no longer be necessary.

Transition:	Increase vegetable and fruit consumption
	One meal each day of vegetables only
	Additional servings of fruit
Supplementation:	Reduce, and ultimately eliminate Plant enzymes

IDEAL DIET

The Ideal Diet is appropriate for the patient whose urine and saliva pH readings indicate his body is functioning normally and maintaining an adequate alkaline reserve. This diet consists of 75% fruits and vegetables, 30% of which should be eaten raw, and 25% grains, nuts, seeds, and, if desired, meat, fish or poultry. Plant enzymes can be taken with a meal even on this diet.

Ideal:	75% Fruits and Vegetables (30% raw)
	25% Grains, nuts, seeds, meat, fish, poultry
	No processed, synthetic, or stimulatory substances

Breakfast should be a meal of fruit; the mid-day meal, a starch meal; and the evening meal should be the protein meal. Listed below are examples of specific fruit, starch, and protein meals.

Fruit Meals

1. Orange and grapefruit

2. Orange and pineapple

3. Grapefruit and sour apples

4. Banana, pear, dates, sweet grapes

5. Figs, dates, sweet grapes, sweet apples

Starch Meals

1. Vegetable salad, carrots, potatoes, beets

2. Vegetable salad, okra, brown rice, cauliflower

3. Vegetable salad, green squash, fresh corn, asparagus

4. Vegetable salad, squash, okra, whole grain bread

5. Vegetable salad, broccoli, chard, yams

Protein Meals

1. Vegetable salad, green squash, spinach, nuts

2. Vegetable salad, yellow squash, cabbage, sunflower seeds

3. Vegetable salad, okra, green beans, cottage cheese

4. Vegetable salad, turnip greens, broccoli, eggs

5. Vegetable salad, green squash, green beans, roast beef (if desired)

(Vegetable salad is a combination of any non-starch vegetables)

GUIDELINES FOR HEALTHFUL MEALS

Eat only when hungry.

Eat food that nature made — not food that man made. Eat the food as nearly as possible the way nature made it, not overcooked or processed.

Eat some raw foods at every meal.

    Breakfast - Eat fruit
    Mid-day   - Eat a starch meal
    Evening   - Eat a protein meal

After eating a fruit meal, wait one hour before eating food from another food group.

After eating a starch meal, wait two hours before eating food from another food group.

After eating a protein meal, wait three hours before eating food from another food group.

<u>Foods to be Avoided</u>

Processed foods or synthetic foods should not be included in any diet, nor should the items in the following lists be used; they should be eliminated from the diet slowly — one at a time.

Coffee	Salt	Fried Foods
Tea, Stimulants	Herb Teas	Margarine
Carbonated Beverages	Spices	Milk
Kool Aid		

Processed meats	White Sugar, White Flour
Ham, Bacon	Pies, Cookies, Cakes
Hot Dogs, Salami	Macaroni, Spaghetti
Bologna	Crackers
	Ice Cream

When all of these foods have been eliminated, the patient will be ready to begin on the Ideal Diet.

QUALITY OF FOODS

Patients who have progressed to the Ideal Diet will want to know more about what constitutes "good" food. Some of the qualities they can look for as they select their menus are:

1. Wholeness. Food should be as nearly complete and as close as possible to the form it was when it came from the garden or tree. Avoid fragmented, processed, or "instant" foods.

2. Rawness. Although it is difficult to eat raw food exclusively, we can, with relative ease, eat about 30% of our daily consumption raw. This amount will give the body material which it can use to make enzymes to digest the remainder of the foods. Spinach should always be eaten raw.

3. Ash. The food should have an alkaline ash. Fruits and vegetables, with the few notable exceptions of cranberries, rhubarb and plums, satisfy this requirement.

4. Quantity. Patients will be less inclined to overeat if they confine their diets to fruits and vegetables. Good food is usually self-limiting, however, it is possible to overdo — as with any excess, overeating should be avoided.

5. Compatibility. Even good foods can have adverse effects if they are improperly combined at a meal. Never eat protein and starch at the same meal, and always eat melon alone.

Make sure that food is combined in such a way that it does not act as a "poison" to the body. The more sick a person is, the more important proper food combining becomes and the more important it is to eat only one food at a meal. (See Food Combining Chart, p. 173.)

MONITORING AND ANALYSIS SYNOPSIS

The chart shown on page 183 is designed for the patient to record his urine and saliva pH levels in a form that will provide both the doctor and patient a comprehensive picture of progress. The pertinent data supplied by the patient is used to evaluate pH levels. In order to assess the patient's condition from pH level readings, it is essential to know the food that was consumed the previous night and the number of hours the patient slept before the first morning urine sample; test paper used to determine the pH of urine cannot differentiate between an alkaline reaction due to ammonia or bicarbonate and an alkaline reaction due to alkalizing minerals.

The last column, "How I Feel," gives the doctor vital information for drawing conclusions as to the extent of the patient's alkaline reserve. In this column, the patient can keep a daily record of particular symptoms that may be pertinent in determining how his diet should be altered. The chart below is a summary of findings after a meat or vegetable meal.

FINDINGS AFTER A MEAT MEAL

Urine pH	Symptoms	Recommendation
Below 6	Stiffness	Distilled water - 2 qt. p/day
Above 6	Stiffness	Cranberry juice - 2 qt. p/day
Above 6	Bladder pain	Nothing to eat EXCEPT Cranberry juice - 3 qt. p/day

Note: (1) Urine pH below 6 is equally as toxic as pH above 6 caused by ammonia and bicarbonate, however, it is not as painful.

(2) The patient should discontinue smoking, drinking coffee or cola drinks, and eating candy during this time. If these activities are continued, the body will respond much more slowly.

FINDINGS AFTER A VEGETABLE MEAL

Urine pH	Response
Below 6	The body is using all of the neutralizing substances available, leaving an acid urine.
Above 6	1. The body's alkaline reserve is adequately supplied and the excess fixed alkaline substances, sodium, calcium, and potassium, are being eliminated directly into urine.
	2. The body does not have the ability to digest vegetables, consequently, the alkalizing substances are not absorbed, pass directly into the urine, and give a false high pH reading.
	3. May be due to emotional stress of a sick patient. Acid is being produced despite good food, resulting in ammonia in the urine. Restless sleep is often a part of the pattern that produces an ammonia urine after a meal of vegetables.

Chiropractic care is an important part of the program to restore the patient to health. All dietary recommendations are made assuming that the patient is being adjusted with B.E.S.T. as he improves his nutrition habits. By using the B.E.S.T. system, the patient's body can utilize both the food and the supplementation to the maximum degree. Physiological timing is improved with each B.E.S.T. adjustment allowing digestion to improve and maximum health to be recovered.

Anything that is eaten — good or bad — represents an emergency situation to which the body must respond. The body cannot ignore substances that are put into it; it will either process the substances normally or eliminate them. Both of these processes take the body's energy and attention. Food is a priority that creates "stress" — either good or bad. During restful sleep, the body's digestive processes break down complex materials while anabolic processes repair and replenish cells. The waste material that is not usable, for whatever reason, is then eliminated. As a result of this anabolic activity, the readings of the first urine specimen of the morning provide the doctor with two very important pieces of information. <u>First</u>, it tells how the body reacted to yesterday's food intake; and, <u>second</u>, it provides an indication of the availability of vital reserves of the body when a controlled diet is followed.

Saliva pH should not be affected by the food the patient ate the night before. Saliva pH is an indicator of intracellular condition, particularly the cells of the liver. Emotional states, unsettling or stimulatory dreams, or restless sleep can result in abnormally high first-morning saliva pH readings. By obtaining an accurate patient history as well as dietary information, the doctor is better able to evaluate the patient's condition. The patient who agrees he must change his diet but prefers to continue to eat meat should consume only enough fruits and vegetables to raise the urine pH one unit higher than the saliva pH, i.e., saliva pH 5, urine pH 6.

A patient whose diet consists of a high percentage of meat may have a saliva pH of 5 and urine pH of 7. If this person suddenly begins to eat large quantities of fruits and vegetables, he may be subject to bladder infections resulting from the abrupt change in urine pH. This condition will generally clear up in a few days if the patient drinks several glasses of cranberry juice per day. Cranberry juice is one of a very few fruit juices that have an acidifying effect on the body. More severe dietary changes may be in order to improve the pH readings of a more seriously ill patient. It may be necessary for him to give up all animal protein and limit protein-rich grains and beans to one serving per day.

A word of caution: Any time cranberry juice is recommended, it is important that the patient understand that this in only a temporary measure. Cranberry juice should never be consumed on a regular basis; its only purpose is to acidify the body quickly in order to provide symptomatic relief. Cranberry juice contains aromatic acids that are not metabolized by the body. These acids remain intact throughout the entire digestive process, acidifying the urine and bladder as it exits the body.

A period of time is required after altering eating habits for the digestive system to readjust to normal physiology and function. To accommodate to the more healthful diet, betaine hydrochloride with enzymes will help the digestive system of a very toxic patient through the period when the body's digestive system is being restored to normal.

FOOD COMBINING

STARCH

Molasses	+2507.1	Barley, Perled	– 21.3
Brown Sugar	+1440.	Chocolate Cake	– 18.8
Dried Beans	+ 282.3	White Flour	– 26.5
Dried Limas	+ 123.	Whole Wheat Flour	– 26.4
White Potatoes	+ 26.3	Brown Rice	– 28.7
Ice Cream	+ .4	White Bread	– 28.8
Cookies	+ or –	Macaroni/Spaghetti	– 50.
Corn Syrup	0	Peanuts	– 78.
Granulated Sugar	0	Peanut Butter	– 80.3
Corn Oil	0	Oatmeal	– 95.
Olive Oil	0	Soda Crackers	– 104.4
Honey	– 4.4	Dried Lentils	– 171.4
Fresh Corn	– 8.8	Wheat Germ (1T.)	– 37.7
Whole Wheat Bread	– 14.5	Wheat Bran (1T.)	– 10.4

SWEET FRUIT

Dried Figs	+297.
Dried Dates	+ 80.7
Bananas	+ 17.9
Raisins	
Prunes	
Avocado	+ 44.

VEGETABLES—SALADS

Spinach	+556.2
Beet Greens	+447.9
Celery	+341.25
Chard Leaves	+214.4
Water Cress	+192.
Sauerkraut	+176.1
Lettuce	+170.8
Green Limas	+142.8
Cucumbers	+142.8
Radishes	+129.8
Rhubarb	+116.5
Cabbage	+110.6
Broccoli	+101.4
Beets	+ 97.9
Brussel Sprouts	+ 94.6
Carrots	+ 93.6
Green Soy Beans	+ 85.
Parsnips	+ 67.2
Rutabegas	+ 62.1
Cauliflower	+ 50.9
Mushroom	+ 49.6
Green Beans	+ 38.9
Onions	+ 14.4
Green Peas	+ 4.6
Fresh Corn	– 8.8
Tomato	+

MELONS

Muskmelon	+ 37.5
Watermelon	+ 5.32

DAIRY

Yogurt
Eggs (See Protein)
Milk
Cheese
Butter
Ice Cream
    (See Starch List)

PROTEIN

Eggs	– 9.
Pork Chops	– 9.9
Lamb	– 17.
Lamb Chops	– 17.
Turkey	– 23.4
Beef	– 24.3
Veal	– 37.2
Chicken	– 43.4
Corned Beef	– 79.7
Bacon	– 94.27
Sausage	–160.7
Dried Beans	+282.3
Dried Lima	+123.
Dried Soy Beans	+ 80.5
Dried Peas	+ 57.5
Dried Lentils	–171.4
Shrimp	– 4.
Salmon	– 26.3
Codfish	– 51.26
Haddock	– 77.62
Sardines	–160.6
Oysters	–209.6
Scallops	–226.2
Almonds	+274.3
Brazil Nuts	+115.7
Peanuts	– 78.
English Walnuts	–100.3
Peanut Butter	– 80.3

ACID FRUIT

Limes	+33.
Cherries, Sour	+30.15
Tangerines	+29.15
Strawberries	+27.5
Grapefruit	+25.2
Lemons	+23.5
Pineapple	
Oranges	+21.8
Grapes	+10.
Plums	–
Cranberries	

SEMI ACID

Apricots	+25
Blackberries	+22.8
Peaches	+21.2
Raspberries	+18.6
Pears	+ 9.6
Blueberries	+ 4.9
Apples	+ 4.7

Food Combining Chart compiled from material in: (1) Herbert M. Shelton, *Food Combining Made Easy* (San Antonio, Texas: Dr. Shelton's Health School, 1976). (2) Dr. R.A. Richardson, *Strong, Healthy Eyes Without Glasses* (Kansas City, Missouri: The Eyesight and Health Association, 1925). (3) Charles D. Hodgman, M.S., ed., *Handbook of Chemistry and Physics* (Cleveland, Ohio: Chemical Rubber Publishing Co., 1959). (4) Maynard A. Joslyn, ed., *Methods in Food Analysis, 2nd Ed.* (New York and London: Academic Press, 1970). (5) F. Leslie Hart, A.M., and Harry Johnstone Fisher, Ph.D., *Modern Food Analysis* (New York: Springer-Verlag, New York, Inc., 1971).

14

QUICK REFERENCE REVIEW

Urinalysis can provide the most current information on the health status of patients. Blood tests can reveal how the body has responded to past diet, stress, trauma, and life style; urinalysis can indicate how the body is functioning on a day-to-day basis.

This chapter is a distillation of the information presented in the preceding chapters. It can serve as a ready-reference for the various facets of urinalysis, physiology, and biochemistry that have been discussed in more detail elsewhere in this book.

One of the tools for analyzing patients' urine is the composite reagent strip that reacts to elements of and in the urine, such as pH, protein, glucose, ketones, bilirubin, blood, nitrites, and urobilinogen. These and other aspects of urinalysis are addressed synoptically in the following pages for your use as a reference aid.

ASCORBIC ACID

Ascorbic acid, or vitamin C, in the urine indicates that the patient is getting an adequate amount of this vitamin and is eliminating the excess.

BILIRUBIN

Bilirubin is a direct register of liver function.

Bilirubin is a product of the breakdown of red blood cells. Bilirubin in the urine indicates that the liver is unable to function correctly and the kidney is acting as a detoxification back-up system.

Bilirubin should not appear in the urine in any amount.

Urine pH will usually be acid when bilirubin is present.

Bilirubin in urine of pH 8 may indicate a serious condition.

Specific gravity may be elevated when bilirubin is present.

Short-term fasting and long-term changes in nutrition habits will allow the body to detoxify. Changes in the toxicity level can be monitored by bilirubin readings.

Initial treatment for bilirubin in the urine is a 24-hour water fast. Following the water fast, a juice fast will allow the body to cleanse itself of accumulated toxins — fresh carrot juice and fresh fruit juice are preferable.

The liver may lose up to 70% of its functioning capacity before symptoms become apparent.

In rapid cleansing when large quantities of juice are consumed (especially carrot juice) the liver may not be able to accommodate to the volume of toxins released for elimination; these toxic substances will cause the skin to turn yellow, but the stools will retain normal color.

Jaundice

Types and signs of jaundice:

Hemolytic — yellow eyes; bilirubin not present in urine

Obstructive — yellow eyes; bilirubin present in urine

Dietary — white eyes; bilirubin not present in urine

Dietary changes are always necessary in treating jaundice.

The most important indicator of the progress of the jaundice condition is the whites of the eyes. If the whites retain their clear white color and the skin yellows, the body is cleansing, and improvement is likely.

If a patient comes to you with yellowing skin but the whites of the eyes are still white, he should begin a 24-hour water fast followed by the institution of cooked vegetables or soups, and then progress slowly to raw vegetables.

If the whites of the eyes turn yellow as the skin turns yellow and bilirubin appears in the urine, the patient is in a critical condition. If a patient in this condition is on a cleansing fast, he should immediately begin to eat cooked vegetables.

BLOOD

Blood in the urine is very significant. A patient who has blood in the urine must be checked every day.

Blood in the urine will be in one of two forms: whole red blood cells, or hemolyzed.

Whole red blood cells originate from a rupture somewhere in the body. The rupture may be in the glomerulus, or the rupture could be the result of a trauma or torn blood vessels as a result of too much protein.

When excessive RBC destruction is indicated, anemia should be considered.

Hemolyzed blood indicates a greater destruction of red blood cells than the liver can handle.

The patient should consume nothing but cranberry juice until there is no longer blood in the urine. If there is a large quantity of blood or if the condition continues for more than 48 hours, the patient should be referred to another care provider for further investigation.

CLARITY OF URINE

Urine should be clear — transparent — not cloudy.

Cloudy urine can indicate a kidney infection.

Urine may become cloudy from either phosphates or pus. The primary cause of cloudiness is phosphates that are insoluble in an alkaline urine.

If the pH is 7.0 or above, phosphates should be suspected. To differentiate between phosphates and pus, after all tests have been completed with the urine sample, let it sit for 5-10 minutes. If pus or mucous is causing the cloudiness, it will settle to the bottom and a division of urine and contamination will be visible to the naked eye.

If this settling does not occur, add a teaspoonful of vinegar (distilled or cider) to the urine sample. If it remains cloudy, mucous or pus is the cause; if it clears, phosphates are the cause.

COLOR OF URINE

In a healthy patient, urine is ordinarily is straw to amber in color.

B vitamins will give urine a bright yellow color.

Urine other than straw to amber in color, could be the result of the patient taking prescription drugs for a bladder infection, or of the use of recreational drugs.

> *Medication for a bladder infection is aimed at neutralizing the ammonia in the urine. This can be accomplished equally as well by having the patient drink two to four glasses of cranberry juice a day, or by having him drink one teaspoonsful of distilled vinegar in a glass of water three times a day.*

Distilled vinegar for a bladder infection is a short-term procedure only. Distilled vinegar is detrimental to health, however, it helps to relieve the symptoms of a bladder infection.

Distilled vinegar is a pure acetic acid that leaves no alkaline ash. The quantity of acetic acid is so great that it will not all be metabolized. The remainder passes into the urine where it acidifies the urine and neutralizes the ammonia that causes burning on urination. Apple cider vinegar will not effect the symptomatic relief that distilled vinegar does since it has not been distilled and retains the alkaline-ash producing properties.

When urine is red or brown in color, blood should be suspected. If blood in the urine is confirmed, further investigation is necessary to determine the source of the bleeding.

GLUCOSE

Glucose is a normal substance in the blood but can appear in abnormal concentrations. When the concentration is too high, the kidney cannot process all of it and the extraneous glucose is eliminated in the urine.

Glucose can be high after consuming substantial amounts of maple syrup, honey, or fruit.

Glucose in the urine could indicate toxicity rather than an insulin deficiency exclusively — most diabetics have adequate or excess amounts of insulin in their blood.

Approximately 75% of glucose is stored in the liver, and approximately 25% is stored in other cells. Unlike glucose in the liver, glucose in muscle cells cannot be released for use in other functions of the body.

INDICAN

Indican in the urine indicates significant toxicity. An end product stemming from insufficient secretion of pancreatic enzymes, indican is more indicative of the condition of the colon than of the level of pH.

Indican is a result of incomplete protein digestion in general and incomplete processing of the protein amino acid tryptophan in particular due to inadequate secretion of a pancreatic enzyme. When tryptophan is in the large intestine, it putrefies into indole. Indole is a highly toxic substance that is converted into indican in the liver. The indican then enters the bloodstream, is filtered out of the blood in the kidney, but is not reclaimed and returned to the blood; consequently, it passes out of the kidney in the urine and is excreted.

When indican is present in the urine, it is a signal that the body needs help in digesting protein. Treatment including reduction of protein consumption and enzymatic supplementation that includes betaine hydrochloride will eliminate the indican from the urine in 21 days.

Indican in the urine indicates an extreme degree of toxicity that can be associated with migraine. The indican level can be monitored as an indicator of progress of the detoxification program of a patient who suffers from migraine.

KETONES

Ketone readings should be negative.

Vitamin C can mask ketones in the urine. Patients who consume large amounts of fruits or vitamin C supplements may show a false negative ketone level.

Ketones are a form of energy that can be used by the body, i.e., brain cells.

> *During a fast, the patient is burning excess stored fuel and not suffering starvation. During a fast, if ketones disappear from the urine for 48 hours and hunger is constant, the fast must be terminated since starvation will follow.*

> *The preferred fast is one of only vegetable or fruit juice until the first phases of ketosis is reached and the urine pH is 6.1. As long as ketones are present and the urine pH is 6.1 or above, diabetic (or acidotic) coma will not occur.*

Ketones plus bilirubin may indicate cleansing is taking place too fast.

In the cleansing process, there should never be more than a trace of ketones.

> *During cleansing, the ketone level can be regulated by the amount of carbohydrates consumed. An average size man performing a minimal amount of exercise (such as walking 2-3 miles per day) can consume as much as two or three bananas per day to maintain a trace during the cleansing process. More food than this will bring the patient out of ketosis and provide nutrients for germs or disease; less food than this will put the patient in too high a level of ketosis.*

> *A fasting patient who shows high levels of ketones must be supervised closely by daily monitoring for signs of bilirubin. (See Bilirubin in this chapter)*

NITRITES

Nitrites indicate the presence of bacteria in the bladder that are reducing nitrates from the diet to nitrites.

Treat with cranberry juice or distilled vinegar until the nitrites are no longer present.

ODOR

Urine should be odorless.

If urine has fruity or acetone odor, diabetes, fasting, or dehydration should be suspected. This odor may also be apparent after the patient has eaten asparagus or garlic, or has taken drugs.

Most urine samples will have an odor of ammonia and a high pH reading, and the patient may be experiencing bladder irritation.

When the ammonia odor is present but the urine pH reading is not 6.4 or above, the patient will probably not have symptoms of a bladder irritation. This is an indication that too much protein has been consumed in the past and that the patient will likely experience symptoms of disease in the future if his eating habits are not altered to replenish the alkaline reserve that is being diminished.

pH and pK

pH Values

0.00 – 6.99   = acid

7.00   = neutral

7.01 – 14.00 = alkaline

MONITORING AND ANALYSIS SYNOPSIS

Recommended Meal Sequence for Evaluating Toxicity

For the Week of _____

	URINE pH				SALIVA pH						
Date	No. Hours Sleep	Meal Previous Night	pH First Sample A.M.	First pH on Arising	5 min. After Breakfast	Before Evening Meal	After Evening Meal	Before Lemon Test	2 min. After Lemon Test	How I Feel
		Regular Meal								
		Meat Meal								
		Meat Meal								
		Regular Meal								
		Vegetable and Fruit Meal								
		Vegetable and Fruit Meal								
		Regular Meal								

MEAT MEAL   After 5:30 pm, drink only water and eat your choice of ONLY steak, pork, fish, fowl, bread, pasta, beans.

VEGETABLE MEAL   After 5:30 pm, drink only water and eat LARGE QUANTITIES of only potatoes, green beans, zucchini, broccoli, celery, carrots.

1. Number of Sleep Hours are those of continuous sound, uninterrupted sleep.
2. First Saliva pH is taken before brushing teeth, preparing or even thinking about food.
3. Breakfast should be about 30 minutes after first Saliva pH.
4. Lemon Test: Check saliva pH after having had no food for at least two hours. Squeeze the juice of 1/2 lemon into glass of water and drink mixture. Check saliva pH again after 2 minutes.

pK of Buffering Systems		Optimum pK of
Bicarbonate Buffer System	6.1	Extracellular fluid
Phosphate Buffer System	6.8	Intracellular fluid
Protein Buffer System	7.4	Blood

Saliva pH generally follows pattern of urine pH, however saliva rises at a much slower rate than urine pH.

High protein diet + alkaline urine + acid saliva = kidneys unable to reabsorb neutralizing minerals; alkaline reserve depleted.

High vegetable diet + acid urine + acid saliva = low alkaline reserve; alkalizing minerals being retained to neutralize acids.

Urine pH

Urine pH can range from 4.5 to 8.5.

Almost all literature that addresses the question of urine pH is written as though acid urine were normal. However, an acid urine pH is not normal, it is necessary. This condition is so pervasive in people who are asymptomatic that it appears to be standard. Urine pH readings give the most current, accurate information on the body's capability to handle the food that has been consumed within the past day.

Monitoring the pH of the first voiding of the morning indicates how the body is responding to food eaten the day before. The reagent strip will show a high pH reading if (1) ammonia and bicarbonate are present in the urine, or (2) there is sodium, calcium, or potassium in the urine. The pH readings must be evaluated in conjunction with the foods eaten within the past 12 hours.

Upon arising, urine and saliva readings of 6.8 pH or above following an evening meal of vegetables, fruits, and only alkaline-ash producing foods, indicate the alkaline reserve is sufficient to allow additional neutralizing elements of sodium, calcium, and potassium to be eliminated. If the saliva pH read-

IMPLICATIONS OF *URINE* pH READINGS

MEAL BEFORE SLEEP	pH 1ST SPECIMEN A.M.	CAUSE	CORRECTION
ACID ASH	4.5 to 5.8	Too much dietary protein. Losing sodium fast but alkaline reserve still available to produce acid salt.	TRANSITIONAL DIET. Have patient eat as usual adding one vegetable meal per day. Then add one fruit per day. Gradually increase vegetables and fruit. Supplement with: betaine hydrochloride with enzymes—one w/each meal; essence of barley extract; 1 tsp. p/day Egg Calcium.
ACID ASH	5.8 to 6.8	Alkaline reserve very low. Barely able to produce acid urine.	TRANSITIONAL DIET. Change VERY slowly. Supplement with betaine hydrochloride w/enzymes, essence of barley extract, Egg Calcium. May need cranberry juice.
ACID ASH	6.8 to 8.5	Alkaline reserve depleted. Ammonia and bicarbonate pass into urine giving high pH.	MODIFIED DIET. Use caution in changing diet. Subject to bladder irritation if high alkaline ash foods instituted even if some meat is eaten. For bladder irritation or infection, put patient on up to two quarts per day of ONLY cranberry, cranapple, or cranraspberry juice for two days. Supplement with betaine hydrochloride with enzymes, essence of barley extract, Egg Calcium.
ALKALINE ASH	4.5 to 5.5	Organic minerals from alkaline foods going directly to cells. No alkaline reserve built.	TRANSITIONAL DIET. pH will rise slowly with increase in amount of vegetable and fruit eaten and demands of cells satisfied.
ALKALINE ASH	6.8 to 8.5	Two Possibilities: **1.** Everything Normal or	**1.** IDEAL DIET if saliva pH 6.8 or better consistently and patient is asymtomatic.
		2. Cells so toxic cannot use alkaline minerals of food. Increased supplementation and Modified Diet immediately.	**2.** MODIFIED DIET. Supplement with essence of barley extract 1 tsp p/day increasing to 3 tsp p/day.

ing is below 6.1 and the urine pH reading is 6.8 or above, the body is so toxic that the minerals cannot be absorbed from the blood into the cells and are passing through the digestive tract.

A urine pH of 6.8 or above following an acid-ash producing meal indicates that the body is so toxic that the alkaline reserve is depleted and ammonia and bicarbonate are being eliminated in the urine giving a false alkaline reading.

Urine pH will usually be acid when bilirubin is present.

Urine pH of 8 with bilirubin present may indicate a serious condition.

Saliva pH

Saliva pH gives an indication of the intracellular environment and is the most accurate indicator of overall health and the condition of the alkaline reserve. The lemon test demonstrates the availability of buffering substances.

LEMON TEST

Check saliva pH two hours after eating.

Squeeze juice of one-half lemon into a glass of water. Drink the mixture, recheck saliva pH after two minutes and note change.

Saliva pH should be consistently 6.8 pH (the pK of the phosphate buffer system) or higher. Saliva pH readings should never be below 6.1, the pK of the bicarbonate buffer system.

Saliva pH below 6.1 indicates the body is acid and the alkaline reserve is inadequate to handle the acid of additional acid-ash producing foods.

Patients whose saliva pH is under 6.1 should not engage in strenuous physical activity, such as jogging, that causes cells to produce additional acid.

IMPLICATIONS OF *SALIVA* pH READINGS

pH BEFORE MEAL	pH AFTER MEAL	CAUSE	CORRECTION
5.8 or Below	5.5 or Lower than Before Meal	Worst scenario: Patient sick for so long, cells too toxic to function. Body cannot use alkalizing food. Patient constantly moving; foot-bouncer. Sleeps only 2–3 hrs. at a time, never deep sleep. Tendency to use drugs. May take 6 months correction before patient "feels good"; may take year for ideal pH values.	MODIFIED DIET. Supplement with betaine hydrochloride with enzymes, essence of barley extract. May need cranberry juice. Change diet slowly. As diet improves, pH readings slowly rise after first meal of day.
5.8	5.8	pH stays the same rather than going down after meal; shows alkaline reserve is improving.	Gradual shift to TRANSITIONAL DIET. Monitor saliva and urine pH readings. Gradually add more vegetables and fruits as readings improve. Continue supplementation until pH readings in "Ideal" range.

Essence of barley extract should be continued for those who eat out or travel frequently. |
5.8	6.2	Alkaline reserves continue to improve. Body regaining control. Bicarbonate buffer system working and diet improvement can increase. Eating causes only minimal physiological pH response.	
6.2	6.8	Minimum pathophysiological involvement. Should improve rapidly.	
6.8	6.8	Body under control. More improvement noted. Bicarbonate and phosphate buffers working.	
6.8	6.8–7.0	*Restless. Unable to sleep soundly.* May show high pH erroneously as body operates under emergency physiological response.	MODIFIED DIET. Person has much stress in life that must be dealt with before pH will respond in favorable manner.
6.8	6.8	Normal physiological functions. Asymptomatic, able to sleep six hours.	This patient can be on IDEAL diet.

LEMON TEST: Check saliva pH two hours after eating. Squeeze juice of one-half lemon into glass of water. Drink mixture, check saliva pH again after 2 minutes and note change.

PROTEIN

The most common protein in urine is albumin.

Protein in the urine may indicate (1) a kidney infection, heart failure, or liver disease, or (2) excess protein has been consumed and is being eliminated as waste.

The patient who has been on a high-protein diet for a period of time and, as a result, has become highly toxic will eliminate protein and ammonia in the urine.

This patient may not express dramatic symptoms. However, his overall state of health has deteriorated and it will be only a matter of time until he experiences the symptoms of chronic degenerative disease.

Immediate but gradual modification of diet is called for to begin to replenish the alkaline reserve.

Kidneys will back up the liver in the detoxification process. Kidney cells break down protein as best they can, but if there is more protein than the kidney can handle, the protein will be dumped directly into the urine.

Excess protein can be toxic to the liver.

SPECIFIC GRAVITY

Specific gravity of 1.015 - 1.025 is considered normal for urine.

Specific gravity of 1.030 indicates the patient is not drinking enough water. Elevated specific gravity can also be due to protein in the urine.

Specific gravity of 1.005 indicates the patient may:

    (1) be drinking large volumes of water,

    (2) drink large quantities of coffee or tea,

    (3) have just consumed a large portion of watermelon, or

(4) be eliminating unconcentrated urine with no reabsorption properties due to the pituitary gland secreting inadequate amounts of an anti-diuretic hormone.

Only water is excreted when the kidneys lose the ability to act as a purifier. The cells of the glomerulus can become so congested that they cannot absorb the waste materials from the blood to be eliminated in the urine.

When bilirubin is present, urine specific gravity may be elevated and the urine may be dark (yellow-green) in color.

Specific gravity readings should return to normal as the patient's dietary habits and health improve.

UROBILINOGEN

Urobilinogen in the urine is considered by some to be normal, however, urobilinogen may be evidence that the body is toxic.

Urobilinogen may be an indication that increased red blood cell destruction is taking place faster than the body can adequately process it and that a toxic condition exists in the colon.

BRIEF NOTES AND REMINDERS

Physiological toxicity is the first step toward chronic degenerative disease.

Vegetarians can eat alkaline-ash producing foods exclusively and still be acid as a result of negative thinking.

A cold is a cleansing process; the body has reached its saturation point and the body is "dumping" toxic substances through all exits. Orange juice exacerbates the cleansing. Cranberry juice for 24 - 48 hours will alleviate symptoms — cranberry juice neutralizes ammonia.

Chronic degenerative diseases are "rescue remedies" — they are accommodations by the body to conditions imposed on it. If the body had not made the necessary adaptations that resulted in the development of the chronic degenerative disease, the patient would have long since died from excess toxicity. A carrot juice fast supplemented with one to three glasses of cranberry juice daily will neutralize the toxicity-generating acid.

Allergic reactions or morning stiffness can be the result of eating alkaline-ash producing food which contributes to an environment already alkaline due to ammonia. Patients who experience these symptoms should not consume powerful alkalizers such as citrus or tomatoes — green beans and squash will rebuild their alkaline reserves more slowly and allow them to accommodate to acids and preclude further problems.

Distilled vinegar is devoid of minerals; the alkaline-ash producing properties have been extracted.

Apple cider vinegar retains alkaline-ash producing properties.

Food is a stimulant. Physiological stimulation to maintain homeostasis should be regulated internally by the endocrine system rather than externally by consuming stimulatory substances such as drugs, caffeine, meat, chocolate, or sugar.

The body has the ability to produce acid — it has an endless supply of acidifying substances, including the acid produced by cells in their normal functioning. The body has no supply of alkalizing substances except bicarbonate that must have sodium, calcium, potassium, magnesium, or other collaborating minerals to perform its alkalizing function.

There is no such thing as metabolic alkalosis except as extreme acidosis.

WARNING: The Standard American Diet may be harmful to your patients' health.

AFTERWORD

This book has been written in response to the many requests of doctors who have attended my lectures on nutrition. As doctors, we all are constantly looking for ways to help our patients improve their health and to live longer, more vital, pain-free lives. My experience has shown that by understanding urinalysis and utilizing the concepts set forth in this book, doctors can guide their patients toward both immediate and long-term rewards of improved health. I hope that the practicing doctor will find this information helpful in clarifying (both for himself and his patients) some of the hitherto confusing results of urinalysis.

Many of the principles and concepts put forth here are the result of looking at old truths in new ways. It is my sincere hope that this information will enable you to serve more effectively those patients who come to you for assistance.

I welcome your comments concerning your experiences in using the methods described in this book as well as any suggestions of ways this material would be of more benefit to you. I will consider this book a resounding success and my efforts and time in producing it well spent if it stimulates additional research and analysis of the premises presented here. My greatest expectation is to spur the academic and scientific communities to approach these hypotheses with a true sense of intellectual exploration that will refute or reinforce my findings.

M.T. Morter, Jr., B.S., M.A., D.C.
101 Pleasant Ridge Lane
Rogers, AR 72756

REFERENCE NOTES

CHAPTER ONE: INTRODUCTION

1. "Dietary Goals for the United States," Prepared by the Staff of the Select Committee on Nutrition and Human Needs, United States Senate, (Washington, D.C.: U.S. Government Printing Office), February 1977, p. v.

2. Ibid., p. 13

3. "Dietary Goals for the United States," Prepared by the Staff of the Select Committee on Nutrition and Human Needs, United States Senate, (Washington, D.C.: U.S. Government Printing Office), December 1977.

4. "Dietary Goals for the United States,"   February, op. cit. p. 6.

CHAPTER TWO: CONCEPTS AND ASSUMPTIONS

1. Arthur C. Guyton, M.D., *Textbook of Medical Physiology*, 2nd ed., (Philadelphia and London: W.B. Saunders Company, 1961), p. 111.

2. Abraham Cantarow, M.D., and Bernard Schepartz, Ph.D., *Biochemistry*, (Philadelphia and London: W.B. Saunders Company, 1954), p. 267.

3. K.C. Cole, "Is There Such a Thing as Scientific Objectivity?" *Discover* (September 1985): pp. 98-99.

4. D.W. Martin, P.A. Mayes, V.W. Rodwell, *Harper's Review of Biochemistry*, 18th ed., (Los Altos, Calif.: Lange Medical Publications, 1981), p.273.

5. John A. McDougall, M.D., Mary A. McDougall, *The McDougall Plan*, (Piscataway, N.J.: New Century Publishers, Inc., 1983), p. 103.

CHAPTER THREE: IMPLICATIONS OF pH IN URINALYSIS

1. George A. Wilson, D.C., D.Sc., FCBRS, FICC, *The 2nd Factor in Chiropractic: Including Proteinoid and Carbonoid Urine Tests for Nutrition and Body Poisons*, Second ed., (Standard Research Laboraties, 1959), p. 86.

2. Arthur C. Guyton, M.D., *Textbook of Medical Physiology*, 2nd ed., (Philadelphia and London: W.B. Saunders Company, 1961), pp. 125-126.

3. Guyton, op. cit., p. 838.

4. Charles D. Hodgman, M.S., Robert C. Weast, Ph.D., Samuel M. Selby, Ph.D., *Handbook of Chemistry and Physics*, 40th ed., (Cleveland, Ohio: Chemical Rubber Publishing Co., 1958), p. 1721.

5. Abraham Cantarow, M.D., Bernard Schepartz, Ph.D., *Biochemistry*, (Philadelphia and London: W.B. Saunders Company, 1954), p. 267.

6. Guyton, op. cit., p.111.

7. Irwin M. Arias, M.D., David Schachter, M.D., Hans Popper, M.D., David A. Shafritz, M.D., *The Liver Biology and Pathobiology*, (New York: Raven Press, 1982) p. 555.

8. W.W. Tuttle, Ph.D., Sc.D., Byron A. Schottelius, Ph.D., *Textbook of Physiology*, 14th ed., (St. Louis: The C.V. Mosby Company, 1961), p. 309.

9. Guyton, loc. cit.

10. Guyton, 7th edition, p. 441.

11. Guyton, op. cit., p. 442

12. Tuttle, op. cit., p. 113.

CHAPTER FIVE: THE ROLES OF ACID AND ALKALI IN THE BODY

1. D.C. Jarvis, M.D., *Arthritis and Folk Medicine* (New York: Fawcett Crest, 1960), pp. 68-69.

CHAPTER SIX: URINALYSIS INDICATORS

1. Arthur C. Guyton, M.D., *Textbook of Medical Physiology*, 2nd ed., (Philadelphia and London: W.B. Saunders Company, 1961), p. 154.

2. Casey Horton, ed. *Atlas of Anatomy*, (Secaucus N.J.: Chartwell Books, Inc., 1985), p. 118.

3. Irwin M. Arias, M.D., David Schachter, M.D., Hans Popper, M.D., David A. Shafritz, M.D., *The Liver Biology and Pathobiology*, (New York: Raven Press, 1982) p. 438.

4. Guyton, op. cit., p. 971.

5. Clayton L. Thomas, M.D., ed. *Taber's Cyclopedic Medical Dictionary*, Fifteenth Edition, (Philadelphia: F.A. Davis Company, 1985), p. 1291.

6. Hans A. Nieper, M.D., "The Non-Toxic Long-Term Therapy of Cancer: Necessity, State of the Art, Trends," *Journal of I.A.P.M.*, Vol. VI, No. 1: 57.

CHAPTER SEVEN: PROTEIN — EXCESSIVE VS. ESSENTIAL

1. John A. McDougall, M.D., Mary A. McDougall, *The McDougall Plan*, (Piscataway, N.J.: New Century Publishers, Inc., 1983), p. 95.

2. McDougall, loc. cit.

3. McDougall, op. cit., p. 98.

4. Chander Rekha Anand and Hellen M. Linkswiler, "Effect of Protein Intake on Calcium Balance of Young Men Given 500 mg Calcium Daily," *Journal of Nutrition* 404 (1974): 695.

5. Henry G. Bieler, M.D., *Food Is Your Best Medicine*, (New York: Random House Vintage Books Division, 1973), p. 65.

CHAPTER EIGHT: CALCIUM, PROTEIN, AND OSTEOPOROSIS

1. Arther C. Guyton, M.D., *Textbook of Medical Physiology*, Seventh Edition, (Philadelphia: W.B. Saunders Co., 1986), p. 939.

2. Ibid., p. 918.

3. Lindsay N. Allen, Ph.D., E. A. Oddoye, Ph.D., and S. Margen, M.D., "Protein-Induced Hypercalciuria: A Longer Term Study", *American Journal of Clinical Nutrition* 32:741-749 1979, p. 741.

4. Ibid., p. 747.

5. John A. McDougall, M.D., Mary A. McDougall, *The McDougall Plan*, (Piscataway, N.J.: New Century Publishers, Inc., 1983), pp. 52-53.

6. Guyton, op. cit., p. 793.

7. Guyton, op. cit., p. 950.

8. McDougall, op. cit., p. 102.

9. Chander Rekha Anand and Hellen M. Linkswiler, "Effect of Protein Intake on Calcium Balance of Young Men Given 500 mg Calcium Daily," "Journal of Nutrition, 104:695-700 1974, p. 695.

10. Clayton L. Thomas, M.D., ed. *Taber's Cyclopedic Medical Dictionary*, (Philadelphia: F.A. Davis Company, 1985), p. 1291.

11. Guyton, op. cit., pp. 939, 940.

12. Corinne H. Robinson, *Proudfit-Robinson's Normal and Therapeutic Nutrition*, (New York: The McMillan Company, 1967), pp. 343, 344.

13. James M. Orten, M.D., Otto W. Neuhaus, Ph.D., *Human Biochemistry*, Ninth Edition, (Saint Louis: The C.V. Mosby Company, 1975), p. 699.

14. McDougall, op. cit., p. 51.

15. Betty Kamen, Ph.D., and Si Kamen, *Osteoporosis: What It Is, How To Prevent It, How To Stop It*, (New York: Pinnacle Books, 1984), p. 155.

16. Guyton, op. cit., p. 937.

17. Kamen, op. cit., p. 160.

18. Guyton, op. cit., p. 945.

19. Guyton, op. cit., p. 939.

CHAPTER NINE: CHEMICAL REACTIONS IN THE BODY

1. Charles E. Dull, H. Clark Metcalf, John E. Williams, *Modern Chemistry*, (New York: Henry Holt and Company, 1958), p. 67.

2. Therald Moeller, *Inorganic Chemistry: An Advanced Textbook*, (New York: John Wiley & Sons, Inc., 1952), p. 280.

3. Ibid., pp. 284-285.

4. W. Norton Jones, Jr., *General Chemistry*, (New York: The Blakiston Company, Inc., 1954), p. 124.

5. Ibid., Adapted from Activity Series, p. 125.

6. Ibid.

7. Dull, Metcalf, Williams, op. cit., pp. 29, 73.

8. Nuclear Magnetic Resonance of living sodium is different from the sodium found in table salt. These two substances are not interchangeable.

9. Dull, Metcalf, Williams, op. cit., p. 265.

10. Moeller, op. cit., pp. 286-287.

11. Dr. Edward Howell, *Enzyme Nutrition*, (Wayne, NJ: Avery Publishing Group Inc., 1985), p. 3.

12. Ibid., p. 16.

13. Bieler, Henry G., M.D., *Food is Your Best Medicine*, (New York: Random House, Vintage Books Division, 1973), p. 192.

14. Ibid., pp. 197-198.

15. Howell, op. cit., p. 40.

16. Ibid., p. 28.

CHAPTER ELEVEN: ADDITIONAL INDICATORS

1. A.L. Notkins, "Causes of Diabetes," *Scientific American* (November 1979): p. 241.

2. Irwin M. Arias, M.D., David Schachter, M.D., Hans Popper, M.D., David A. Shafritz, M.D., *The Liver Biology and Pathobiology*, (New York: Raven Press, 1982), p. 555.

3. Israel S. Kleiner, Ph.D. and James M. Orten, Ph.D., *Biochemistry*, Sixth ed., (St. Louis: The C.V. Mosby Company, 1962), p. 627.

CHAPTER TWELVE: THE IMPORTANCE OF CORRECT EATING AND EXERCISE

1. James M. Orten, Ph.D., Otto W. Neuhaus, Ph.D., *Human Biochemistry*, (St. Louis: The C.V. Mosbey Company, 1975), p. 488.

2. 100 grams of macaroni = 111 calories; 100 grams of potato baked in skin = 93 calories. Clayton L. Thomas, M.D., M.P.H., ed. *Taber's Cyclopedic Medical Dictionary*, (Philadelphia: F.A. Davis Company, 1985) p. 2060.

3. James F. Fixx, *Jim Fixx's Second Book of Running*, (New York: Random House, 1980), p. 141.

GLOSSARY OF TERMS AS USED IN THIS TEXT

A

acid ash
: Metabolic residue of particular foods, including animal and vegetable protein. Requires buffering, or neutralizing, before being eliminated through the kidneys. Puts additional strain on the body.

acidosis
: High hydrogen ion concentration. The accumulation of more acid in the body than can be handled effectively.

albumin
: Simple proteins found in plant and animal tissue, blood, milk, eggs, and other substances. When albumin is coagulated by heat, it becomes insoluble in water.

alkaline ash
: Metabolic residue of organic foods, including most vegetables and fruits. Can be processed for elimination through the lungs and/or kidneys. Causes little stress to the body.

alkaline reserve
: Substances available to neutralize extra-cellular acid. Stored in cells throughout the body but predominantly in the liver. Made up principally of 1) bicarbonate ions, and 2) fixed reserves of sodium, potassium, calcium, iron, and magnesium.

alkalosis
: Low hydrogen ion concentration. Indicated by high pH readings of urine and saliva. Symptoms similar to acidosis. For persons on a high-protein diet, alkalosis is an advanced degree of acidosis. Ammonia and bicarbonate can be responsible for the condition termed alkalosis.

anabolism	Conversion of nutrients into living tissue.
anaerobic glycolysis	The process of forming adenosine triphosphate (ATP) from glucose when little or no oxygen is available.
ash	Residue of digested food that has been metabolized by the body. May be either acid or alkaline in reaction depending upon the original food of which it is a product.
atom	Smallest part of an element capable of entering into a chemical reaction. Neutral electrical charge.
ATP	Adenosine triphosphate. A high energy compound made from food by the body; found in all cells of the body, particularly muscle cells. Produces high energy when substance is split.
autointoxication	Poisoning by substances produced by the body. Can be normal substances existing in excess amounts.

B

bile	Continuous secretion of liver, stored in gall bladder. Liver bile is straw colored; gall bladder bile is yellow, brown, or green. Bile performs emulsifying action for digestion of fats and oils. Composed of water, bile salts, bilirubin, cholesterol, fatty acids, lecithin, sodium, potassium, calcium, chlorine, and bicarbonate. Normal bile is always alkaline in nature and yellow in color.
bile salts	Alkali salts performing emulsifying or detergent function and as aid in absorption of fatty acids. Absence of bile salts redu-

ces absorption of fat soluble vitamins A, D, E, and K.

bilirubin | Bile pigment produced from biliverdin in the breakdown of hemoglobin in red blood cells. Normal finding in blood; abnormal finding in urine.

biliverdin | A greenish pigment in bile resulting from red blood cell destruction. Biliverdin is reduced to bilirubin.

buffer | A substance that maintains the original hydrogen-ion concentration of a solution when either an acid or base is added.

buffer systems | Bicarbonate, phosphate, and protein buffer systems adjust pH of intracellular and extracellular fluids to pK of environment.

C

candidiasis | Yeast infection of mucous membrane, skin, or nails.

catabolism | Breakdown of complex compounds. Opposite of anabolism.

cholesterol | A monohydric alcohol occurring in a variety of substances, i.e., egg yolk, fats, nerve tissue of the brain and spinal cord, and the liver. Can be synthesized in the liver and is a precursor of various steroid hormones. Highly fat soluble; only slightly water soluble. A normal constituent of bile that is found in most gall stones.

contractive foods | Predominantly acid-ash producing foods. Have a restrictive influence on the body that is characterized by a nervous, intense, high-strung, or violent personality.

contralateral — Affecting opposite sides of the body; simultaneously integrated; crossed.

cooking bonds — Alteration in bonding structure of ions caused by heat.

covalent bonds — Loose chemical link of electrons shared between two atoms. Atoms easily separated, bond easily broken. The type of bond predominant in all living systems.

D

detoxify — Removal of toxic nature of substance.

digestive residue — Waste material from food. Those portions of food that are not metabolized for use by the body. Passes through the small and large intestine and is eliminated through the bowel.

disassociation — Separation of ions of an electrovalent substance during solution process.

E

electrode potential — The degree of ability of an ion to accept or release electrons to become an atom.

electron — Negatively charged particle of atom.

electrovalent bonds — Strong bond between atoms where each accepts from or donates to the other. An ionic link that is not easily broken. The pre-dominant bond of mineral kingdom.

enzymes — Complex proteins capable of producing chemical change in other substances without being altered themselves. Efficiency of enzyme activity can be affected by reaction of medium in which they function.

expansive foods — Predominantly stimulatory substances with little nutritional value and an acidifying ef-

fect on the body. Overindulgence may
produce a sense of euphoria and loss of
ability to concentrate.

extracellular | Outside the cell.

G

glucose | A form of simple sugar. The end product in metabolism of complex carbohydrates.The principal source of energy for the body.

glucosuria | Sugar in the urine.

glycogen | Glucose stored for future use. Animal starch.

glycogenesis | The process of converting excess glucose to glycogen during passage of glucose through the liver.

glycolysis | A process that converts glucose into ATP within the cells. Breaking down of glucose into smaller compounds yielding energy the body can use.

glyconeogenesis | Process taking place in the liver that forms glycogen from noncarbohydrate sources under conditions such as low carbohydrate consumption or starvation. Syn.: gluconeo-genesis

H

homeostasis | Equilibrium or balance of internal environ-ment of the body.

hydroxyl | Commonly referred to as a base or alkali. A radical that can accept one ion of hydrogen and form water.

I

indican	Potassium salt found in urine and sweat, formed by conversion of tryptophan to indole through bacterial action in the intestine then further modified to indican in the liver.
inorganic	Indicates chemical substances other than living entities found in nature.
inorganic acids	Component parts held together by strong electrovalent bonds. Highly ionized; up to 95% of hydrogen ions active at a time. Highly corrosive. Eliminated through excretory system after having been buffered.
intracellular	Within the cell.
ion	Atom or atoms with imbalance of electrons and protons.
ionic bond	Strong, electrovalent bond. Restricts separation of components of substances such as sodium chloride, thereby impeding use of elements by the body.
ionization	The disassociation of acid, base, or salt compounds into their constituent ions. The formation of ions from polar solute molecules by the action of a solvent.
ionization potential	The degree of ability of an atom to gain or lose electrons to become an ion.

J

jaundice	A yellowish tint to the skin often caused by excessive bilirubin in the extracellular fluids.
• dietary jaundice	Non-pathological yellowing of the skin brought about by the consumption of large quantities of carrot juice.

• hemolytic jaundice	Yellowing of skin and eyes resulting from excessive red blood cell destruction occurring at a rate greater than the liver can adequately handle.
• obstructive jaundice	Yellowing of skin and eyes caused by partial or total blockage of bile ducts, or by damage to liver cells.
jejunum	A part of the small intestine, about 8 feet in length, connecting the duodenum and ilium. Important in reabsorption process of bile salts and absorption of nutrients during digestion.
junk food diet	Contemporary diet of many Americans. Consists of high percentage of highly refined carbohydrates, fats, and additives. Processed foods, convenience foods, and fast-food restaurant fare are dominant features.

K

ketones	An organic chemical substance that is an end product of fat metabolism. Found in urine under starvation, diabetic, or rapid cleansing conditions.
ketonuria	Acetone bodies in the urine.
ketosis	Accumulation of large quantities of ketone bodies, including acetoacetic acid, in blood and interstitial fluids. Can be due to starvation or rigid diets devoid of carbohydrates that cause body to metabolize stored fat. Also evident in diabetes mellitus.

L

lysis	Destruction of blood cells by an enzyme.

M

metabolism — Physical and chemical changes within the body transforming nutrients, foods and other substances into usable form.

molecule — The smallest quantity of a chemical substance that can exist independently and maintain its characteristics. Positive and negative charges evenly balanced.

N

nitrates — Salts of nitric acid. May be found in urine after eating bacon or other similarly processed foods.

nitrites — Salts of nitrous acid. When found in urine, may indicate a bladder infection with reducing bacteria present.

O

organic — Indicates chemical compounds containing carbon. Living substances. Covalently bonded.

organic acids — Substances, resulting from the digestion of fruits and vegetables, having component parts held together by loose, covalent bonds. Easily metabolized. Can be eliminated through lungs.

oxidation potential — The relative value of the ease with which an element's electrons move.

P

parietal cells — Large cells of peptic glands that, in the stomach, produce hydrochloric acid that is covalent in nature.

pathology	Abnormal physical conditions produced by disease.
pH	Potential of Hydrogen. Indicates level of acidity or alkalinity of solution. Measured on a scale of 0 – 14 with 7.0 being neutral. The lower the number, the more acid the solution; the higher the number, the more alkaline the solution.
pK	The ionization constant of a solution.
	- of bicarbonate buffer 6.1 - of phosphate buffer 6.8 - of protein buffer 7.4
proton	Positively charged particle of atom.

R

reticuloendothelial cells	Cells of the reticuloendothelial system (RES) that ingest and destroy substances such as bacteria, cell debris, and dust particles.
reverse osmosis water (RO water)	Water purified by filtration of most minerals and impurities through membrane that allows only molecules to pass. More vital than distilled water that has been boiled.

S

Standard American Diet (SAD)	Conventional American diet consisting of the four basic food groups: dairy products, meats, fruits and vegetables, and cereals and grains. Considered by many to be basis of well-balanced meals. Affords excessive amounts of protein.

T

toxic	Resembling poison. Causes stress to the body.

U

urobilin	Brown pigment formed by oxidation of urobilinogen in urine or stools.
urobilinogen	Colorless derivative of bilirubin formed by action of intestinal bacteria. Highly soluble, reabsorbed through intestinal wall into blood to be excreted into urine by kidneys.

INDEX

liver, 25, 53, 54, 60, 65-68, 69, 70,
71, 73, 84, 132, 133, 153,
171, 176, 178, 180, 188
  disease, 123
  intracellular, 137
  ketones, 145
  sugar storage, 144-145
lungs, 31, 32, 36, 40, 56, 57, 58,
80, 83, 102
lymph, 26
magnesium, 57, 107, 112
mastitis, 62
McDougall, John A. and Mary,
95, 101
metabolism, cellular, 17, 20
milk, 45-46, 95, 99-101, 108, 124,
155
  cow's, 86, 99-100
  formula preparations, 100
  goat's, 99-100
  human, 78, 86, 99-100, 104
  pasteurized, 100, 123, 124
  raw, 124, 155
minerals, 43, 84
  covalent, 29, 156-157
  electrovalent, 29
  in water, 155-157
  organic, 134-135, 156-157
mitochondria, 31, 50
molecule, 110, 113
monitoring, 131-141, 148, 168-
172, 184
mononucleosis, 70
multiple sclerosis, 55
muscle, 54, 61, 69, 78, 94, 98,
158, 180
  cramps, 86-87, 106, 162
  recruiting, 161
  re-timing, 160
  soreness, 132
  sugar in cells, 144
Normal, Natural, Necessary, 3, 12,
37, 74, 83, 88, 144
neurological interference, 149
Nieper, Hans A., 73
nitrate, 83, 132, 133
  in urine, 148

nitric acid, 40, 56, 58, 80, 83, 88,
148
nitrites, 148-149, 182
nitrogen, 59, 81, 82, 83, 93
  excretion of, 16, 82
Neuclear Magnetic Resonance, 69
organic, 116
  acid, 56-57, 62, 69, 104
  minerals, 135
organs, 55
osmotic balance, 36, 45, 85, 87, 89,
116
osteoporosis, 45, 84, 86, 89, 91-
108, 117, 124, 131
oxidation, 31, 110, 111-112
  potential, 111
  reduction reaction, 111
oxygen, 30, 57, 110, 114, 115, 156
pain, 160-162
Palmer, D. D., 119
pancreas, 130
  enzymes, 75, 121-123, 125, 127,
128, 135, 164, 180
parietal cells, 27, 29, 59, 81, 135
pH, 3, 11, 25-38, 40, 56, 69, 73-74,
76 77, 79, 80, 87, 102, 109,
117, 121, 123, 126, 164
  bile, 68,
  exercise, 158
  monitoring, 54, 183
  saliva, 21-22, 47, 50, 87, 132,
137-141, 164, 168-171,
184-187
  table, 29
  urine, 12, 21, 47, 50, 63, 77-82,
132-136, 164, 168-171,
184-186
phosphate, 34, 83, 98
  in urine, 178
phosphate buffer system, 32, 33-
34, 35, 36, 37, 54, 80, 103,
137-138
phosphoric acid, 58, 62, 80, 89
phosphorus, 59, 86, 98-102, 104
photosynthesis, 43, 129
pituitary, 145, 189

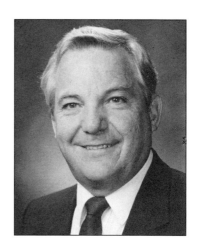

M. T. Morter, Jr.
B.S., M.A., D.C.

Dr. M. T. Morter, Jr., began his investigation into the effects of nutrition on overall health as a result of observing radical differences in the response of his patients to treatment. By applying his scientific background and education to the investigation of nutrition, Dr. Morter has developed a basic method of monitoring and interpreting daily indicators of health.

Dr. Morter earned his academic degrees from Kent State University, Ohio State University, and Logan College of Chiropractic. He has served on numerous professional advisory boards at the state and national levels and is Past President of both Logan and Parker Colleges of Chiropractic.

The work begun in 1972 with the development of the non-forceful procedures of the Bio Energetic Synchronization Technique (B.E.S.T.) has been augmented with nutrition concepts that provide patients with a comprehensive health care program. Since 1965, when Dr. Morter established the Morter Chiropractic Clinic in Rogers, Arkansas, his practice has grown to include 2 clinics, 12 additional doctors and serves over 40,000 patients each year.

In addition to his active practice, Dr. Morter presents technique and nutrition lectures and seminars throughout the United States and worldwide.

The order form below is provided for your convenience in obtaining additional copies of *Correlative Urinalysis* for yourself, your friends, or your associates.

BEST RESEARCH, INC.
1000 W. Poplar
Rogers, AR 72756
1-800-874-1478

Please send _____ copies of *Correlative Urinalysis* to me at

the address below. Enclosed is $_____

Name _____
                                        Print or Type

Mailing Address _____

_____

_____

Cost per copy: $32.00 plus $3.00 shipping and handling
